Leadership and Management Skills for Long-Term Care

Eileen M. Sullivan-Marx, PhD, CRNP, FAAN, RN, is an Associate Professor and Associate Dean for Practice & Community Affairs at the University of Pennsylvania's School of Nursing. She holds the Shearer Endowed Term Chair in Healthy Community Practice. Dr. Sullivan-Marx is an active international and national consultant on nurse practitioner and geriatric practice issues and oversees the School's practice and community mission, which includes the Living Independently For Elders (LIFE), a program of comprehensive integrated health and social services for older adults in West Philadelphia. She is a leading researcher on improving functional outcomes of older adults in community and institutional settings.

Deanna Gray-Miceli, DNSc, APRN, FAANP, is a nationally certified Gerontological Nurse Practitioner with over two decades of experience caring for older adults in academic geriatric practice settings, particularly long-term care, and Adjunct Assistant Professor of Nursing, University of Pennsylvania-School of Nursing. Her program of research includes the development, validation, and feasibility testing of a post-fall assessment tool for RNs and clinical staff to use in the evaluation of older nursing home residents who fall. For the past 2 years, Dr. Gray-Miceli has been a consultant to New York University-John Hartford Institute for Geriatric Nursing (NYU-JHIGN) as Project Director to the JHI/American Association of Colleges of Nursing sponsored grant *"Preparing Nursing Students to Care for Older Adults: Enhancing Gerontology in Senior-Level Undergraduate Courses"* The G-NEC Experience.

Leadership and Management Skills for Long-Term Care

Eileen M. Sullivan-Marx, PhD, CRNP, FAAN, RN
Deanna Gray-Miceli, DNSc, APRN, FAANP

Editors

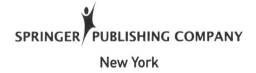

SPRINGER PUBLISHING COMPANY

New York

Springer Publishing Company, LLC
11 West 42nd Street
New York, NY 10036
www.springerpub.com

Acquisitions Editor: Allan Graubard
Production Editor: Julia Rosen
Cover design: Joanne E. Honigman
Composition: Apex CoVantage, LLC

08 09 10 11/ 5 4 3 2 1

Library of Congress Cataloging-in-Publication Data

Leadership and management skills for long-term care / [edited by] Eileen
Sullivan-Marx, Deanna Gray-Miceli.
    p. ; cm.
  Includes bibliographical references and index.
  ISBN 978–0–8261–5993–9 (alk. paper)
 1. Geriatric nursing. 2. Nursing management. 3. Long-term care facilities—
Administration. 4. Nursing services—Administration. I. Sullivan-Marx, Eileen.
II. Gray-Miceli, Deanna.
  [DNLM: 1. Geriatric Nursing—education—United States. 2. Long-Term
Care—organization & administration—United States. 3. Cultural Competency—
organization & administration—United States. 4. Leadership—United States.
5. Patient Care Team—organization & administration—United States.
WY 152 L434 2008]

RC954.L428 2008
618.97′0231—dc22   2007052666

*In memory of our dear friend and
colleague, Lenore H. Kurlowicz, PhD, FAAN,
whose inspiration and dedication will be with us always.*

Contents

Chapter 4

Power and Negotiation 71
Kathleen G. Burke

Chapter 5

Change Theory and Process 97
Linda A. Carrick

Part II: Principles of Education

Chapter 6

Developing Cultural Competence in
Long-Term Care Nursing 121
Rita K. Adeniran and Rosalyn J. Watts

Chapter 7

Leading Through Education in
Long-Term Care Nursing 167
Kathleen L. Egan

Contributors

Rita K. Adeniran, MSN, RN, CMAC, CNAA, BC
Global Ambassador,
Hospital of the University of Pennsylvania
Department of Nursing
Dr NP Student, Drexel University College of Nursing and Health
Professions
Philadelphia, PA

Kathleen G. Burke, RN, PhD
Program Director, Nursing and Health Care Administration and
Health Leadership Masters Programs
Director, Center for Professional Development
School of Nursing
University of Pennsylvania
Philadelphia, PA

Linda A. Carrick, RN, PhD
Kennedy Health System
Vice President, Patient Care Services/Chief Nursing Officer
Voorhees, NJ

Kathleen L. Egan, PhD
Geriatrics Education Consultant/Specialist
Division of Geriatric Medicine
University of Pennsylvania
Philadelphia, PA

Lois K. Evans, PhD, RN, FAAN
van Ameringen Professor in Nursing Excellence
Chair, Family and Community Health Division
Univeristy of Pennsylvania School of Nursing
Philadelphia, PA

Rosalyn J. Watts, EdD, FAAN
Associate Professor Emeritus
Former, Director, Diversity Affairs
School of Nursing
University of Pennsylvania
Philadelphia, PA

Foreword

When I first ventured into long-term care leadership in the early 1980s, I scrambled to find a practical guide to help me with introducing change in organization, structure, planning, staffing, and day-to-day management in the nursing home. There was precious little to be found. So I borrowed ideas and models from hospital and business literature and made my way. Twenty-five years later, however, there *remains* a dearth of practical guides for developing and enhancing nurse leadership in long-term care . . . a place where nursing could and *should* shine. Thus, in settings where stretched resources make effective communication and teamwork imperative to achieve goals, this book is a welcome resource to practicing and aspiring nurse leaders.

The 1980s represented the heyday for the primary nursing model in the acute care arena, but nursing homes still relied on teams of professional and nonprofessional staff to provide a very broad range of services. Fortunately, many long-term care nurses of that era had indeed been educated in team nursing models in their basic programs. Over the years, however, this formal education has been eroded so that, today, there are few professional nurses with formally developed knowledge and skills in leadership and team building. Yet, the team remains the most common model of care in long-term care. Given the dramatic change in acuity and needs of the client population receiving long-term care, such skills are ever more essential for achieving quality of care and quality of resident and work life.

I am very enthusiastic about *Leadership and Management Skills for Long-Term Care* because it brings a rich new resource to nurses and health professionals who care for chronically ill and older adults in long-term care settings. This book fills a long existing gap in the literature, providing information relevant to everyday complex situations requiring team building, leadership, change management, and cultural competence to achieve excellence in geriatric care. Readers can use the book to improve personal understanding in these areas as well as a basis for teaching others in long-term care settings. Ultimately, improving interaction among members of the geriatric care team will be the key to successful and cost effective organizational efforts to change culture, enhance morale, increase nursing staff retention, and improve care.

In the United States, recent funding for a Comprehensive Geriatric Nursing Education program from the Department of Health and Human Services sparked more than 20 projects to support geriatric care and education, one of which provides the basis for this book. Simultaneously, several other exciting and related initiatives have commenced. All are expected to impact quality of care and quality of life in long-term care, and each requires teamwork and professional nurse leadership for change. These include the Geriatric Nursing Leadership Academy funded by a partnership between Sigma Theta Tau International and the John A. Hartford Foundation to train educators and nurse administrators in leadership for care of older adults; a planning project of the five Hartford Centers of Geriatric Nursing Excellence and supported by Atlantic Philanthropies that aims to improve nursing home care through enhancing professional nursing practice in long-term care; and the Hartford Geropsychiatric Nursing Collaborative, which aims to improve the mental health of older Americans, including those in long-term care, through a program of basic, advanced, and continuing education for nurses. This book provides a content resource to these initiatives and can guide faculty and students. Most importantly, the nurses on the front line in long-term care will benefit from this monograph, which was developed for and tested by them and other professionals in similar settings and practices. Thus, the content is fresh and relevant. I know that readers will be heartened by the case studies and straightforward approach used throughout the book. And I believe that readers will find that their own abilities to initiate and manage change for improved long-term care will be enhanced.

—Lois K. Evans, PhD, RN, FAAN
van Ameringen Professor in Nursing Excellence
University of Pennsylvania

Preface

Sometimes the thing staring you in the face is the hardest to see. We refer here to long-term care and the management and leadership skills required to improve care and satisfy caregivers. Discussion of these skills has been sorely lacking in the nursing literature despite the fact that we who provide management and leadership for long-term care have done so, most prominently by "training on the job."

We have written this book to rectify that lack and reflect on the functions we perform and the values we affirm: from clarifying what models of care delivery work best in what situations, to how to best deal with workforce shortages, retention of nursing staff, and sustaining or finding resources to offer competitive salaries for professional nurses.

With funding from the Department of Health and Human Services, Division of Nursing, Comprehensive Geriatric Education, and in partnership with the University of Pennsylvania Geriatric Education Center, we convened a team of experts to develop the educational modules in this book for professional nurses as well as other health professionals in long-term care. All project team members had educational expertise and background in nursing administration and leadership in acute care or clinical expertise in gerontological nursing. Commensurate with what we find currently in the field of long-term care, our team members, who authored these chapters, needed to build expertise across leadership and management for long-term care. As we began the journey, we realized that our nursing administration experts were well informed about leadership and management issues but knew much less about long-term care. Equally, we realized that our gerontological nurse experts were well informed about long-term care but less about leadership and management. As a result, we focused initially on team building and cross-training efforts. Then we developed, tested, and refined the modules in long-term care settings that were both institutional and community based.

Resource experts in educational principles and cultural competence rounded out the team to address the diversity of learning styles, educational backgrounds, and ethnic origins of the staff and older adult residents in long-term care.

Within the chapters in the book, the reader will find a rich resource of leadership and management content and educational principles. Section I, built on some foundational work from a leadership project funded by the Helene Fuld Health Trust, "Forming the Building Blocks of Leadership for Nursing Students Across Academic Levels," includes chapters that cover Team Building, Directing and Delegation in Long-Term Care, Power and Negotiation, and Change Theory and Process. Skills outlined in each chapter provide fresh content and application in long-term care settings that the reader will gain from individually and potentially use for teaching groups. Section II provides key Educational Principles and Cultural Competence content that frames an understanding of successful leadership strategies and how to avoid problems when working in the reality of a rich and diverse environment.

Practitioners, students, faculty, educators, health care executives, nurses and health professionals, employers, and supervisors in long-term care, nursing homes, home care agencies, and home- and community-based programs for long-term care will find the information in these chapters highly relevant and easy to apply in everyday situations. As a whole, this book will fill a long-recognized gap in resources that address the quality of working relationships among nurses and teams in long-term care by providing a resource for skills not commonly or consistently taught in professional education. Using the resources in this book will aid those involved in long-term care in building the entire spectrum of skills required for consistent quality in care, oversight, and management, and in team building and change.

Eileen M. Sullivan-Marx
Deanna Gray-Miceli

Acknowledgments

Funding for this project was provided by Health Resource and Service Administration (HRSA) "Building RN Training Skills for Geriatric Education Excellence," 5-D62HP01912–02–01, E. Sullivan-Marx, PI, the HRSA Delaware Valley Geriatric Education Center, M. A. Forceia and K. Egan, PI; and the Helene Fuld Health Trust, "Forming the Building Blocks of Leadership for Nursing Students Across Academic Levels," J. Thompson, PI.

We wish to express our sincerest appreciation to the following people: Rebecca Phillips, for her commitment and perseverance to direct the project activities and develop teamwork. Sangeeta Bhojwani, for her enthusiasm, valuable organizational skills, and precise formatting work throughout the project and in the final days of submission. Lois Evans, for her inspiration, encouragement, and advice as the project developed and took hold in publication. Maxine Hobson for diligent administrative coordination and support. At the University of Pennsylvania, the Greater Philadelphia Geriatric Education Center and the Hartford Center for Geriatric Nursing Excellence for partnership and colleagueship that ground us all in excellent science and translation to care for older adults. Finally, our team of authors who crossed new frontiers to build knowledge. To our families for their encouragement and love always.

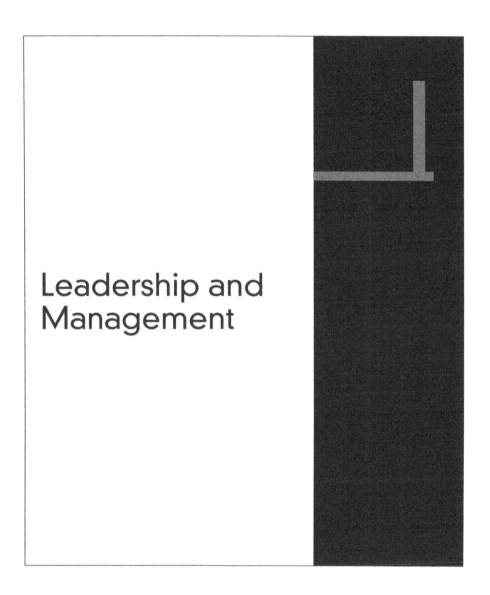

Leadership and Management

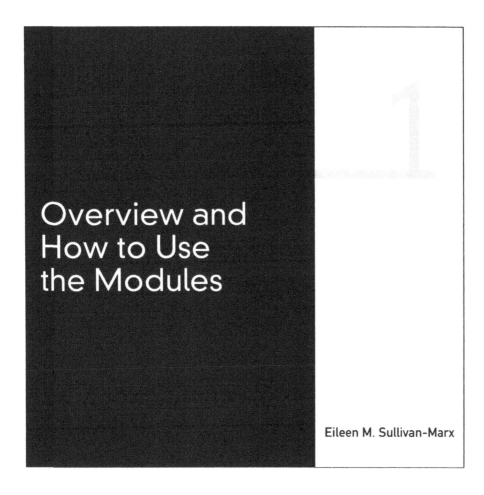

Overview and How to Use the Modules

Eileen M. Sullivan-Marx

Leadership and Management Skills for Long-Term Care was developed to fill a long-recognized gap in training of professional nurses in the requisite leadership and management skills needed in long-term care to improve quality (Jennings, Scalzi, Rodgers, & Keane, 2007). Not commonly or consistently taught in professional nurse training, these skills in leadership, management, cultural competence, and adult education enhance professional nurses' ability to build and interact with the geriatric care team, resolve conflict, negotiate for solutions, develop collaboration, and teach and mentor licensed practical nurses and nursing assistants; they could ultimately be part of a full organizational effort to enhance team morale, improve nursing care of the elderly, and increase retention of all nursing staff.

Not commonly or consistently taught in professional nurse training, these skills in leadership, management, cultural competence, and adult education enhance professional nurses' ability to build and interact with the geriatric care team, resolve conflict, negotiate for solutions, develop collaboration, and teach and mentor licensed practical nurses and nursing assistants; they could ultimately be part of a full organizational effort to enhance team morale, improve nursing care of the elderly, and increase retention of all nursing staff.

The Institute of Medicine (IOM) has highlighted the need for training in leadership to facilitate quality and improve care at the "individual, group, organizational, and interorganizational" levels in health care systems (IOM, 2001, p. 139). To address this need in long-term care and with funding from the Division of Nursing, Health Resources and Service Administration, and the Helene Fuld Trust, we convened a team of experts in health administration, long-term care services, gerontological nursing, cultural competence, and adult education to develop learning modules in leadership and management competencies.

The provision of quality health care to the most frequent users of long-term care, older adults, can be attained when nurses acquire knowledge and skill that carefully follows prescribed educational standards. National accrediting bodies, such as the Association for Gerontology in Higher Education (AGHE), the National League for Nursing (NLN), and the Bureau of Health Professionals, have identified core curriculum and terminal objectives to promote safe and efficacious geriatric nursing practice for entry-level professional nurses. Essential geriatric nursing leadership and management competencies have been developed by the American Association of Colleges of Nursing (AACN) and the John A. Hartford Foundation Institute for Geriatric Nursing (2000). Achieving effective leadership and management within professional nursing practice in long-term care, geared toward an outcome of quality health care for older adults, requires application of 14 core competencies developed in this report.

In each of the chapters, we have carefully outlined examples of how the educational content in the six leadership modules can be used in long-term care practice by professional nurses as they carry out AACN's recommended core competencies for: *Critical Thinking, Communication, Assessment, Technical Skill, Knowledge Related to Health Promotion, Risk Reduction and Disease Prevention, Knowledge Related to Illness and Disease Management, Knowledge Related to Information and Health Care Technologies, Ethics, Human Diversity, Global Health Care, Health Care Systems and Policy, and*

Role Development Related to Provider of Care, Designer/Manager, and Coordinator of Care and Member of a Profession (AACN, 2000).

The provision of quality health care to the most frequent users of long-term care, older adults, can be attained when nurses acquire knowledge and skill that carefully follows prescribed educational standards.

With a team of experts in nursing administration, cultural competence, adult education, and geriatric care, we developed six leadership modules, one on adult education, and one for cultural competence, all specifically focused on long-term care. The expertise of the team chapter authors in each specific area in this text was a major strength of the project. Yet, at the outset of the project it was clear that the experts in nursing administration were less cognizant of long-term care issues, and the geriatric nursing experts were less cognizant of nursing administration issues, a common challenge found both nationally and globally (Aylard, Stolee, Keat, & Johncox, 2003). Before embarking on curriculum development in the area of leadership and management, the project team first self-applied principles of team building and management to coalesce the project working team. We used an inventory of group skills to assess individual and group dynamics as a framework for discussion and project development. All experts had several site visits to the long-term care settings prior to developing the modules and conducting presentations. The project leader who had expertise in both nursing administration and geriatric care brought in one more team member with expertise in both areas to work alongside other team members and bridge areas in which experts identified gaps in perspective or in ways that care is delivered.

A shortage of RNs nationally, particularly in long-term care and home care, impacts the work of LPNs and CNAs because fewer members of the health care team are available to provide care in a coordinated effort. Moreover, the AACN noted in a report by the University of Illinois College of Nursing Institute that "the ratio of potential caregivers to the people most likely to need care, the elderly population, will decrease by 40% between 2010 and 2030" (University of Illinois Nursing Institute, 2001, p. 11). The 2000 IOM study of quality of long-term care recommended addressing nursing aide turnover by improving training,

The AACN notes that "the ratio of potential caregivers to the people most likely to need care, the elderly population, will decrease by 40% between 2010 and 2030."

career development, gaining respect from administrators, clarity of roles, participation in decision making, organizational recognition, and management of workloads.

Why Leadership and Management in Long-Term Care?

Long-term care consists of care provided in traditional nursing homes and community-based settings such as home care agencies or Programs for All-Inclusive Care of the Elderly (PACE), a Medicare-funded program for nursing home-eligible individuals who remain in communities and receive full services through an interdisciplinary team through a capitated financial model. With rising costs and the increasing number of older adults who need long-term care, dynamic changes in long-term care are emerging, requiring nursing staff to have skills to work within organizations that are fluid and yet maintain quality of care. Nursing homes are diversifying their case mix to increasingly care for more acutely ill individuals needing skilled nursing care and acute rehabilitation following hospitalization (Harrington, O'Meara, Kitchener, Simon, & Schnelle, 2003). The challenges for nurses in the area of leadership and management in environments that not only are changing but are emerging and developing in completely new structured models is profound. The need to develop leadership and management skills for nurses in emerging models of long-term care is compounded by the gaps that now exist in these skills for nurses.

This book addresses a long-recognized gap in the quality of working relationships in long-term care by providing RNs with skills not commonly or consistently taught in professional nurse training, namely, leadership, management, cultural competence, and adult education. Building these skills would enhance RNs' ability to teach and mentor LPNs and CNAs and improve interaction with the geriatric care team, and could ultimately be part of a full organizational effort to enhance team morale, improve nursing care of the elderly, and increase retention of all nursing staff (Castle & Engberg, 2006; Werner, 2003).

In 2002, a report prepared by the U.S. Department of Health and Human Services with the Office of Disability, Aging and Long-Term Care Policy and the Institute for the Future of Aging Services identified that the number of nursing assistants in Pennsylvania is expected to grow about 22% between 1998 and 2008, while state projections of need will require a growth rate of about 86% (U.S. Department of Health and Human Services, 2003). More than 50%

of all long-term care providers in Pennsylvania reported staff shortages (Pennsylvania Intra-Governmental Council on Long Term Care, 2002).

Attracting and retaining RNs, LPNs, and CNAs in long-term care of older adults will require creative strategies that promote a positive work environment and improve workers' satisfaction with their ability to care for older adults (Aiken, Clarke, Sloane, Sochalski, & Silber, 2002; Stone et al., 2002). According to the Pennsylvania Intra-Governmental Council on Long Term Care (2002), fewer than half of Pennsylvania's long-term care providers reported increasing participation of CNAs and other direct care providers in care decisions as a strategy to improve retention despite indications of a positive relationship between such worker input and retention. CNAs and LPNs indicated that they have few opportunities for ongoing skill building or professional development in this same study.

In a Report to the Pennsylvania Intra-Governmental Council on Long Term Care (2001) assessing workers' needs in long-term care, CNAs attributed retention problems to the lack of enough nurses and aides to do the work, not enough training, and lack of training that was meaningful to them. Eaton (1997) noted that RNs have little training and skills in how to supervise, motivate, and educate LPNs and CNAs thus contributing to supervision that relies on punitive methods. In contrast, Wellspring Innovative Solutions, Inc. (Wellspring) has managed to decrease staff turnover in long-term care facilities by creating a working environment in which employees have the skills to do their job and a voice in how work should be done, thus enabling team effort. A key facet of success was a commitment and training of RNs to work with and mentor nursing assistants, helping them to apply newly learned skills, and supporting them in decision-making (Stone et al., 2002). This project is consistent with national and state priorities to attract and retain RNs, CNAs, and LPNs in the care of older adults by providing RNs with the skills to teach, lead, motivate, evaluate, and supervise LPNs and CNAs in a culturally competent, sensitive approach to provide excellent geriatric care (AACN, 2000).

As an exemplar to address the need to promote quality of care through leadership for nurses, in 2007, the John A. Hartford

Foundation and Sigma Theta Tau International, the Honor Society of Nursing, initiated a nationwide 18-month mentored leadership experience for aspiring geriatric nurse leaders. The Geriatric Nurse Leadership Academy has been developed through grant funding by the John A. Hartford Foundation and in partnership with the Hartford Foundation's five Centers of Geriatric Nursing Excellence. The purpose of the Academy is to prepare and position nurses in leadership roles in various health care settings to lead multidisciplinary teams in the improvement of health care quality for geriatric patients and their families. Through the multilevel learning activities of the Academy, nurses who have fundamental geriatric knowledge and competence will acquire leadership knowledge and competence that will lead to the improvement of the quality of care and outcomes for geriatric patients. In addition, a nationwide network of geriatric nurse leader mentors will be formalized, and further resources for geriatric nursing leadership and scholarship will be developed.

How to Use This Book

The six leadership modules in this book cover content for (1) Team Building, (2) Communication, (3) Power and Negotiation, (4) Change Theory and Process, (5) Management: Directing and Delegating, and (6) Management: Moving From Conflict to Collaboration. The adult education module focuses on principles of teaching and learning related to adult learning in a clinical environment for care of older adults. The cultural competence module is designed to prepare RNs to incorporate cultural competency as an integral aspect of their practice through appraisal of personal values, beliefs and attitudes about others, impact of racial and ethnic disparities on quality of care, framework for discussions regarding diversity, and concerns of special populations. Several case studies for long-term care have been selected to develop critical thinking skills for adult learners. These modules have been tested in several types of long-term care settings and found to be effective for use by professional nurses, social workers, rehabilitation therapists, and long-term care managers in nursing homes, home care, and community-based long-term care settings.

Funding for this project was provided by Health Resource and Service Administration (HRSA) "Building RN Training Skills for Geriatric Education Excellence," 5-D62HP01912-02-01, E. Sullivan-Marx, PI, the HRSA Delaware Valley Geriatric Education Center,

M. A. Forceia and K. Egan, PI; and the Helene Fuld Health Trust, "Forming the Building Blocks of Leadership for Nursing Students Across Academic Levels," J. Thompson, PI.

We tested the modules at four long-term care settings. Two nursing homes, one a 240-bed federally funded program and another 500-bed city/county funded nursing home; a Program for All-Inclusive Care of the Elderly (PACE) for 250 members; and a large metropolitan home care agency. The sites identified several challenges in their environments that related to the testing of the leadership and management modules. These scenarios are common to all settings in long-term care. The home care agency had a new nursing director who had identified a goal to train clinical nursing supervisors and case managers in leadership and management. The PACE Program had recently experienced a rapid expansion and growth and organizational restructuring. The city nursing home was highly structured with a long-established administrative model that had recently undergone a change in management group and a public relations challenge. The federally funded nursing home had open support from the health system at the executive level and had the highest ratio of RNs to patients than any other site.

The modules presented in this book were presented and tested using pre- and post-test questionnaires and evaluations with 52 registered nurses and a few other health care professionals in the long-term care settings. Of the RNs, 85% were women and 15% were men, which exceeds the national average of men in nursing; 63% were white, 23% black, 9% Latino, and 5% self-described as other. For all four sites, underrepresented minorities comprise approximately 27% of RN staff; in two sites, 40% work with CNAs who are primarily from minority backgrounds and in sites that provide care to underserved minorities with a range of health disparity needs. Modules were presented separately at sites and revised based on questionnaires and evaluations. At a final half-day conference, the project team, participants, and administrators presented and responded to findings and lessons learned.

Challenges for the sites and project team in providing training to long-term care sites were the mounting staff pressures and job demands along with tight schedules, which prevent consistent participation in training and on-site education. Long-term care sites do not always have technology for educational materials, such as power point and computer LCDs, or budgets to support accommodations

Long-term care sites do not always have technology for educational materials, such as power point and computer LCDs, or budgets to support accommodations and refreshments for their participants. Scheduling on-site participation for educational sessions can be interrupted by staff shortages, health department survey visits, severe weather, faculty availability, or other situational problems.

and refreshments for their participants. Scheduling on-site participation for educational sessions can be interrupted by staff shortages, health department survey visits, severe weather, faculty availability, or other situational problems. Therefore, this book can provide resources that can be used as self-learning tools or as tools to teach others with power point slides or handouts as appropriate to setting. Digital supplements containing the power point slides, and the tests and participant evaluation forms in the text are easily accessible via the Springer Publishing Company Web site (www.springerpub.com). Click on the link and type in the password, Sullmarx.

This book is written for the self-learner as well as for trainers who would use the modules for group training. Each module chapter is structured to provide a pre- and post-test, learning objectives, topical content, case studies, handouts, and evaluation. The individual learner can take the pre-test for the chapter content and following review of the content in the chapter as well as the power point handout, take the post-test to gauge improvement as well as areas needed to review. The educator who uses the book for group training can give the participants the pre-test. Following the pre-test, the educator can use the chapter content to create discussion and/or lecture and use the power point slides as visual aids for the lecture content or for content review by group participants. Following completion of each chapter, the group participants can take a post-test. Results from the post-test can be shared with individual participants to ascertain their achievement as well as identify learning needs. The answers to the tests can be found in the Appendix. Results from the post-test can be aggregated by the educator to recommend review of content for the participants and highlight need for further training. Finally, the evaluation form could be distributed to group participants to provide feedback to the educator or educators regarding how the session achieved goals as well as steps for improvement in subsequent sessions.

References

Aiken, L. H., Clarke, S. P., Sloane, D., Sochalski, J., & Silber, J. H. (2002). Hospital nurse staffing and patient mortality, nurse burnout, and job dissatisfaction. *Journal of the American Medical Association, 288,* 1987–1993.

American Association of Colleges of Nursing (AACN), The John A. Hartford Foundation Institute for Geriatric Nursing. (2000). *Older adults: Recommended baccalaureate competencies and curricular guidelines for geriatric nursing care.* Washington, DC: Author.

Aylard, S., Stolee, P., Keat, N., & Johncox, V. (2003). Effectiveness of continuing education in long-term care: A literature review. *The Gerontologist, 43,* 259–271.

Castle, N. G., & Engberg, J. (2006). Organizational characteristics associated with staff turnover in nursing homes. *The Gerontologist, 46,* 62–73.

Eaton, S. C. (1997). *Pennsylvania's nursing homes: Promoting quality care and quality jobs.* Keystone Research Center High Road Industry Series, #1. Harrisburg, PA.

Harrington, C., O'Meara, J., Kitchener, M., Simon, L. P., & Schnelle, J. F. (2003). Designing a report card for nursing facilities: What information is needed and why. *The Gerontologist, 43,* 47–57.

Institute of Medicine. (2001). *Crossing the quality chasm: A new health system for the 21st Century.* Washington, DC: National Academy Press.

Jennings, B. M., Scalzi, C. C., Rodgers, J. D., & Keane, A. (2007). Differentiating nursing leadership and management competencies. *Nursing Outlook, 55,* 169–175.

Pennsylvania Intra-Governmental Council on Long Term Care. (2001, February). *In their own words: Pennsylvania's frontline workers in long term care.* Report to the Pennsylvania Intra-Governmental Council on Long Term Care. Author: Harrisburg, PA.

Pennsylvania Intra-Governmental Council on Long Term Care. (2002, October). *In their own words: Part II.* Report to the Pennsylvania Intra-Governmental Council on Long Term Care. Author: Harrisburg, PA.

Stone, R. I., Reinhard, S. C., Bowers, B., Zimmerman, D., Phillips, C. D., Hawes, C., et al. (2002). *Evaluation of the Wellspring model for improving nursing home quality.* Institute for the Future of Aging Services & the American Association of Homes and Services for the Aging. New York: The Commonwealth Fund.

University of Illinois Nursing Institute. (2001). *Who will care for each of us? America's coming health care labor crisis.* Author: Chicago, IL.

U.S. Department of Health and Human Services. (2003). *State-based initiatives to improve the recruitment and retention of the paraprofessional long-term care workforce.* Retrieved January 22, 2008, from http://aspe.hhs.gov/daltcp/reports/pltcwf.htm

Werner, J. M. (2003). An assessment of strategies for improving quality of care in nursing homes. *The Gerontologist, 43,* 19–27.

Team Building

Pre-test (circle one)

Please circle the *best* answer among the items listed below.

Example:

This is a test.

   a.   No, this is not a test.
   (b.) Yes, this is a test.
   c.   No, this is a joke.

The answer is (b) so it will be circled.

1. Senn, Childress, and Senn describe four styles of behavior in their self-scoring behavioral style/instrument. Which style is not described by this inventory?

   a.   Controlling
   b.   Promoting
   c.   Judging
   d.   Analyzing

2. There are many characteristics of effective teamwork. What is the major requirement for effective teamwork?

   a.   Respect
   b.   Openness
   c.   Empowerment
   d.   Trust

3. A team is

   a.   An individual who is working on his/her own to accomplish a goal
   b.   A group of people who are independent of each other but work to achieve a common group goal
   c.   A group of people who are dependent on one another to achieve a common goal
   d.   None of the above

4. When working with someone with a controlling style, all of the following behaviors are effective EXCEPT:

   a. Spend time on the relationship before jumping to the task
   b. Make your presentation stimulating and exciting
   c. Be decisive and self-confident
   d. Let them do most of the talking

5. Describe your behavioral style. (2 points)
6. Identify the strengths and weaknesses of your style. (4 points)

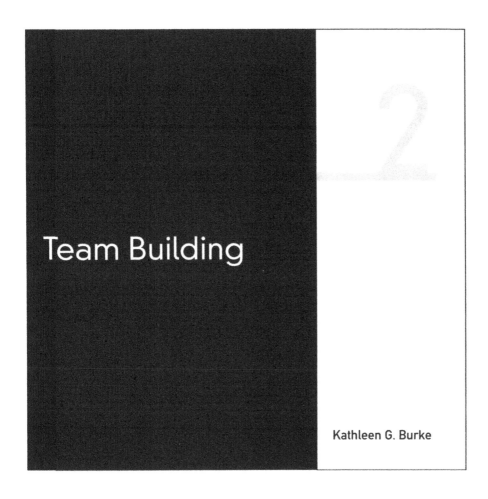

Team Building

Kathleen G. Burke

Individual commitment to a group effort—that is what makes a
team work, a company work, a society work, a civilization work.
—Vince Lombardi

Teams and teamwork are important components of the delivery of
health care. Patient care always involves input from members of
different professions who work together to coordinate care across
multiple settings and during various stages of health and illness.
Coordination of care is an essential element of geriatric care, especially in light of the looming incidence of chronic illness and associated comorbidities experienced by older adults, especially those
in long-term care. The ability to communicate and work together is
essential for continuity and safe patient care, especially if medical

errors are to be eliminated. Effective administrative managers in health care organizations understand and are able to evaluate the skills and overall strength of different team members, matching them with jobs that are consistent with their strengths and abilities. When team members are composed of such individuals, it is likely that the overall team will be cohesive in unity and thus capable of collaborating effectively in the delivery of health care.

Purpose

The purpose of this chapter on team building is to help nurse leaders understand more about other members of the team as well as their own personal attributes so as to build better relationships and more effective teams within the health care workplace. In this chapter, we will discuss the advantages and disadvantages of working on teams and learn how to work more effectively on teams by first assessing our own, and others, behavioral styles.

Objectives

By the end of this chapter you will be able to:

- Describe the advantages and disadvantages of working on a team.
- Describe your typical behaviors as a team member using the behavioral inventory assessment tool (Senn, Childress, & Senn, 2000).
- Discuss the importance of understanding the strengths and weaknesses of different behavioral styles to improve team effectiveness.
- Develop a plan to capitalize on your strengths.
- Create a plan to address your developmental needs.
- Identify how effective teams/members implement AACN essential competencies for geriatric health care.

Definition

A team is a group of people who are mutually dependent on one another to achieve a common group goal. Teams form in the workplace through administrative assignment or appointment, and some change from day to day depending on the staffing level and other administrative concerns, such as the level of patient acuity.

For example, in the long-term care setting, the medical director and director of nursing colead or direct others in the team for the delivery of effective health care to older adults. Individual team members include licensed and unlicensed personnel ranging from nurses' aides, physical therapists, nutritionists, and registered nurses. Typically a team leader is identified to work with others toward achievement of common group goals. Teams are administratively responsible to current federal regulations and state health policy.

Advantages, as well as disadvantages, occur when working on a team (see Table 2.1 and Table 2.2). Advantages could be development of relationships, increased shared information, or better development of ideas. Disadvantages include logistical scheduling problems, additional time to build the team, and longer time to reach a decision.

Often teams are task specific, and as a result there are trade-offs, or pros and cons, that can occur among any of the associated personal or behavioral characteristics or communication. For instance, consider in the practice setting the creation of a new team to be assembled for patient safety consisting of all members of patient care. At first, individual team members do not know all the

2.1 Twelve Advantages of Working in Teams

- More input leads to better ideas and decisions
- Higher quality output
- Involvement of everyone in the process
- Increased ownership and buy-in by members
- Higher likelihood of implementation of new ideas
- Widens the circle of communication
- Increased learning with shared information
- Increased understanding of other people's perspectives
- Increased opportunity to draw on individual strengths
- Ability to compensate for individual weaknesses
- Provides a sense of security
- Develops personal relationships

2.2 Twelve Disadvantages of Working in Teams

- Requires more time
- Can lead to many meetings
- Often difficult to schedule mutual time
- Requires individuals to give more of themselves
- May take longer to make a decision
- May be used as an excuse for a lack of individual effort
- Personality conflicts are magnified
- Disagreements can cause strained relationships
- Potential for subgroups to form
- Teams can become exclusive rather than inclusive
- May lead to unclear roles
- "Group think" can limit innovation

rules and regulations governing patient safety law and the sanctions imposed that are translated into working policy in the institution. While an advantage is that everyone on the unit (the patient care team) is involved, and buy-in is likely, in reality, team meetings to learn all of the rules take so much time, are complex and overwhelming, and team members can get discouraged and disinterested in participation if a specialty role for each team member is not developed. This can lead to ineffective teams.

Selective Perception

Team effectiveness is complex and dependent upon many factors. One's ability to communicate and work together cohesively on a team depends on our understanding of behavior—ours and other team members. Our past experiences, values, beliefs, and interests all shape our worldview to create our *selective perception filter* (Senn, Childress, & Senn, 2000). We continually evaluate people and situations through this selective filter. We tend to either lock-in or lock-out things in the perceptual awareness of our environment. For example, look at the Figures 2.1 and 2.2. A critical question is to ask yourself: "what do you see in the first picture?"

2.1

Perceptual
Illusion: Young
Woman/Old
Woman

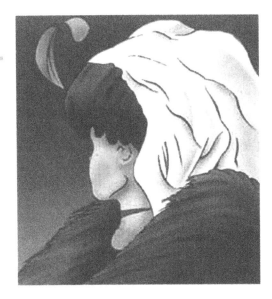

2.2

Perceptual
Illusion: Young
Woman/Skull

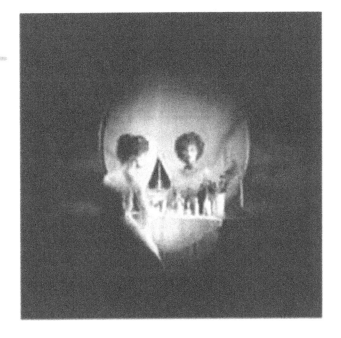

In Figure 2.1, people may initially see an old woman, but other people may see a beautiful young woman. If you tend to see the old woman first, you probably will have to force yourself to see the young woman. In Figure 2.2, most people initially see a scary-looking face of a skull. But if you look closely, you will see the image of a beautiful Victorian young woman looking at herself in the mirror. In daily life, we have a tendency to do a similar kind of lock-in or lock-out due to our perceptual awareness and resulting inclination to "see" only what our *selective perception* has conditioned us to see (Senn, Childress, & Senn, 2000). We all see the world differently. When we think about this example in relation to teams, team members, and how they function, we can see the relevance. Overall, our individual and unique *selective perception* influences our ability to communicate and work with each other on a team. So, when we think about teams and how they are or are not functioning in the delivery of health care, we must first critically think about each others perceptual awareness: what is it? how to elicit it? And then lastly, how to construct communication effectively so as to individually teach/reach each member of the team.

Behavioral Style Inventory for Teamwork

If you want to interact effectively with me, to influence me . . . you first need to understand me.

—*Stephen R. Covey*

Because of selective perception and lock-in/lock-out, we see the world differently and therefore develop our own unique style. Problems arise, however, when we assume that people see the world the same way we do; if their style is different than ours, we assume there is something wrong with them (Senn, Childress, & Senn, 2000). It is difficult to work as a team unless we appreciate the uniqueness of each person's style. Often times, in order to understand the world from differing points of view, guidance can be obtained from tools, such as the behavioral style framework. It offers us a tool that builds on our strengths and works on our own weaknesses. Further, it helps us understand the strengths and weaknesses of others and helps us avoid judgments, improve communications, and gain more respect for the differences of others.

Characteristics of Behavioral Styles

The four behavioral styles developed by Senn-Delaney Inc. addressed on this tool include: Controlling, Supporting, Promoting, and Analyzing (Senn, Childress, & Senn, 2000). Most people display elements of each style at different times. However, people tend to prefer one style and can generally be identified by the characteristics of that style. The following descriptions give you a brief picture of the four major behavioral styles.

Controlling Style

The controlling style places a big importance on goals and results. These people tend to like being in charge; they are strong willed, forceful, and work with a sense of urgency. They are seen as competent and determined, task oriented, business-like, and they are usually not looked to for encouragement or support. Their approach to work is focused on *results*. They are willing to confront others; they are decisive, concerned with efficiency, and typically their drive for results limits their ability to cooperate and build a team.

The controlling style places a big importance on goals and results. These people tend to like being in charge; they are strong willed, forceful, and work with a sense of urgency.

The challenges of working with this behavioral style is that they can be offensive to others, autocratic, insensitive, impatient, over-controlling, poor listeners, and poor delegators. When you analyze your own behavioral style, critically ask: Does this describe your behavioral style? And can you think of someone that you work with on your team who has elements of controlling style? If yes, how have you handled working with this type of behavioral style in the past?

A general management strategy when working with a controlling behavioral style is for you to adapt your working style by: (1) getting to the point in a discussion, (2) being specific, and (3) keeping the conversation focused on business. Do not waste time. Speak and act quickly. Provide options for them to choose and an overview, but have details available if needed. Overall, be decisive and self-confident, and always let them make the final decision.

Supporting Style

The supporting style's main concern is relationships and the feelings of others. They are loyal, likeable, understanding, cooperative, willing to be of service, patient, and often also empathetic. In general, the supporting style's approach to work is that they are strong team builders, good at reconciling factions that might be in conflict, and able to build quality relationships to get the job done. They tend to want to create win–win solutions versus a competitive approach. They are likeable, inoffensive, and usually don't impose on others. Although this style sounds like a perfect style for team effectiveness, beware; there are challenges with this style.

> The supporting style's main concern is relationships and the feelings of others. They are loyal, likeable, understanding, cooperative, willing to be of service, patient, and often also empathetic.

The supporting style has a hard time confronting marginal performers, and they give in to more dominant personalities. Because they are not demanding enough and need approval, they don't always get the results that are needed for the team. This behavioral style needs to be more results focused and to stand up for their ideas.

A general management approach when working with a supporting style is to: (1) show sincere interest in them and their feelings, (2) be cooperative rather than pushy, (3) be patient, (4) draw out their ideas and concerns, (5) gently explore areas of disagreement, and (6) avoid open conflict. In general, it is helpful to be encouraging and build their confidence by spending time on your relationship with them before jumping into a particular task.

Supporting style people tend to be good listeners who take time with people and help them relax and to be at ease. Do you think you have a supporting style? Do your coworkers demonstrate elements of this style? How do you think your team would function if all its members were a supportive style?

Promoting Style

The main focus of the promoting style is *excitement* and activity. They tend to be energetic and get excited easily. They are creative and get bored easily, enjoying new and varied challenges.

The promoting style's approach to teamwork includes motivating and inspiring others. They express their ideas and opinions persuasively, and they are quick decision makers. But, they can easily change their decisions if they aren't working. They require minimal structure in order to maximize creativity.

The challenges of working with the promoting style is that they tend to exaggerate, and they start more things than they can finish. They often settle for less than the best in order to move on to the next exciting challenge, and they jump to conclusions too rapidly. They are poor at planning and follow-through.

Follow these general management strategies when adapting your style to working with the promoting style: (1) allow time for exploring mutually exciting possibilities, (2) let them do most of the talking, (3) avoid arguing, rather, look for alternative solutions, (4) try and look at the big picture and avoid bogging them down with details, and (5) make your presentation stimulating and exciting, and be open to their ideas.

The promoting style tends to get involved in active, rapidly moving situations. They are lively, personable, and stimulating to be around. Do you have a promoting style? Can you identify someone you know that has a promoting style? Do you like working with them? What do you find most challenging?

> The promoting style's approach to teamwork includes motivating and inspiring others. They express their ideas and opinions persuasively, and they are quick decision makers. But, they can easily change their decisions if they aren't working. They require minimal structure in order to maximize creativity.

Analyzing Style

The analyzing style tends to like structure and order. They have good planning skills and are conscientious, persistent, and steady. The analyzing style is good at follow-through and at setting up systems and structure.

The analyzing style's approach to work is that their first step in problem solving is to gather information. They tend to be cautious in decision making and rarely make big mistakes. They are relied on by others to maintain standards. They study and analyze before making a decision, and they make decisions based on factual information.

The challenges in working with the analyzing style are that they are *risk-averse* and overly cautious. They tend to procrastinate to avoid mistakes. They mistrust their feelings and intuitions and can be indecisive. The

> The challenges in working with the analyzing style are that they are *risk-averse* and overly cautious. They tend to procrastinate to avoid mistakes. They mistrust their feelings and intuitions and can be indecisive. The analyzing style becomes paralyzed and avoids taking action because of their need for data. Under stress they become noncommunicative and withdrawn.

analyzing style becomes paralyzed and avoids taking action because of their need for data. Under stress they become noncommunicative and withdrawn.

In general, some management strategies to work more effectively with the analyzing style are: (1) avoid giving them surprises, (2) be patient, (3) cover each item thoroughly, and (4) be organized and logical. Try to avoid hype (if you have a promoting style). Give them time to get comfortable with the situation, and ask their help in finding the facts and minimizing the risks.

Can you think of someone on your unit that has an analyzing style? This person is usually the person that everyone on the unit relies on to know the policy and procedures. They seem to be the "anchor of reality" because of their logical manner and their thorough approach to problem solving. Do you think you have the characteristics of the analyzing style?

In sum, there are four major behavioral styles, each with unique characteristics. As you form new teams in health care, it is helpful to analyze behavioral characteristics of potential team members and make appropriate selections accordingly. In general, managers will strive for balance with minimal conflicting behavioral styles when forming new teams. If conflicts do arise with the team, team leaders are charged with identifying and resolving these issues. Successful teamwork is contingent on a blend and balance of behavioral styles geared toward achieving a common goal.

Conclusion

Working on a team requires an understanding of each team member's strengths and weaknesses and an appreciation of the contributions of each person. The behavioral style framework helps us better understand ourselves and others and how to adapt our behaviors and communication to the needs of our teams (Senn, Childress, & Senn, 2000). The three most important words in effective teamwork are *trust, trust,* and *trust.* In order to trust and be trusted, we must be tolerant of differences, respectful of other's opinions, willing to compromise, and aware that not everyone thinks like we do. Learning to understand different behavioral styles leads to better understanding and to trust (see Table 2.3). Teams are an important component of the delivery of efficient and effective health care for all people. In Table 2.3 we highlight areas for geriatric care that can be especially relevant for care of older adults who rely on teams in long-term care to deliver coordinated and continuous types of health care.

	Application of AACN's Geriatric Competencies to Assist in Effective Team Building in Long-Term Care

2.3

AACN Competency:	Goals and critical questions to ask:
1. Critical Thinking:	<u>Goals</u>: Recognize one's own and other's attitudes, values, and expectations about aging and their impact on care of older adults and their families; adopt the concept of individualized care as the standard of practice with older adults. <u>Examples of some critical questions to ask:</u> A. What is the selective perception filter of the health care organization? Of the team leader? Of team members and other support staff? B. Do team members view old age positively? Negatively? And how does this view influence the function of the team, if at all? C. Do team leaders and members acknowledge individualized care as the standard of practice?
2. Communication:	<u>Goals</u>: Communicate effectively, respectfully, and compassionately with older adults and their families; recognize the biopsychosocial, functional, and spiritual changes of old age. <u>Examples of some critical questions to ask:</u> A. How do team members communicate within teams and between teams? *1. What is the process?* - Is communication verbal or written or both? - Does it carry a positive intonation or is it overtly critical? - Is communication goal-oriented? Patient-centered? Age-appropriate? - Is communication flawed by issues related to likes or dislikes of team members? - Is communication regular at set intervals or on demand when patient care problems arise?

(Continued)

AACN Competency:	Goals and critical questions to ask:
2. Communication (Continued)	2. *What behavioral styles do team members demonstrate, and how can you effectively communicate given these styles? (For example, are team members controlling? supporting?)* 3. *What is the process for identifying a break-down in communication?* How is it identified? Who is involved? Has it influenced the older adults' satisfaction with care management? 4. *How is communication failure managed?* - Does a change in policy or practice occur? - Does the change in procedure result in improvement in communication? If so, how do you know? - Are older adults and/or their families apprised of communication problems and their solutions? B. Does the team communicate directly with the older adult or family caregiver, if so, are age-appropriate teaching methods incorporated? 1. *What are the methods of communication?* Is communication verbal, or are written instructions in large bold print provided? 2. *Does the team acknowledge each older adult's style of learning or readiness for behavioral change?* 3. *Is the speed of delivery of the message altered for older adults with cognitive or sensory impairment?* 4. *Are team recommendations tailored to the older adult who might experience sensory deficits, such as visual or hearing loss?* (for example, reduction of background noise due to presbycusis; use of large and bold printed materials for visual impairment)

(Continued)

AACN Competency:	Goals and critical questions to ask:
2. Communication (Continued)	*5. How is communication delivered to the older adult with transitory stages of cognitive impairment due to delirium or for those with dementia?* *6. Is adequate time allotted for older adult's feedback and discussion?*

3. Assessment:	<u>Goals</u>: Incorporate into daily practice use of valid and reliable tools to assess biopsychosocial, functional, and spiritual status; assess the older adults' living environment with special awareness of their biopsychosocial and functional status; analyze community resource effectiveness for maintaining functional independence; assess family knowledge of skills needed to deliver care to older adults.
	
	<u>Examples of some critical questions to ask</u>:
	
	A. Is the team performing a clinical assessment of the older adult?
	  1. If so, do they utilize and communicate results from standard empirically tested measures of geriatric health, function, cognition, psychological, and social function?
	  2. Do clinical assessments consider cultural issues?
	  3. Are team members skilled in geriatric assessment? If not, are opportunities for continuing education provided?
	  4. Do teams include or outsource advanced-practice nurses and experts in geriatric care?
	B. What are the processes for communicating the results of the assessment to the older adult?

4. Technical Skill:	<u>Goals</u>: Adapt technical skills to meet the functional, biopsychosocial, and endurance capabilities of older adults; individualize care and prevent morbidity and mortality associated with the use of physical and chemical restraints in older adults.

(Continued)

AACN Competency:	Goals and critical questions to ask:
4. Technical Skill (Continued)	A. Do team leaders and staff possess knowledge and technical skill that is age-appropriate? For instance, are they aware of the age-related factors influencing the assessment and presentation of vital signs? Of physical assessment findings? B. Do team leaders and staff possess knowledge of the harmful effects of physical or chemical restraints in an older adult? Can they identify appropriate behavioral intervention without use of physical or chemical restraint? C. Is care individualized for older adults within the health care organization? If so, how is this measured?
5. Core Knowledge:	<u>Goals</u>: Prevent or reduce common risk factors that contribute to functional decline, health promotion, risk reduction, impaired quality of life, excess disability in older adults; follow standards of care disease prevention to recognize and report elder mistreatment; apply evidence-based standards to reduce risk, screen, immunize, and promote healthy lifestyles in older adults. <u>Examples of some critical questions to ask</u>: A. Do health care providers and team members seek to identify risk factors for functional decline, geriatric syndromes (for instance, urinary incontinence, falls, and pressure sores?), polypharmacy, or elder abuse? Are plans of care individualized?
6. Core Knowledge: Illness and Disease Management	<u>Goals</u>: Recognize and manage geriatric syndromes common to older adults; recognize the complex interaction of acute and chronic comorbidities common to older adults.

(Continued)

AACN Competency:	Goals and critical questions to ask:
6. Core Knowledge: Illness and Disease Management (Continued)	<u>Examples of some critical questions to ask:</u> A. Do health care providers utilize national recommendations and clinical practice guidelines in their assessment and management of various health conditions affecting older adults? Is there overlap among various team members in assessment? B. If so, are these guidelines referred to in the clinical practice protocols?
7. Core Knowledge: Information and Health Care Technology	<u>Goals</u>: Use of technology to enhance older adults' function, independence, and safety; facilitate communication through transitions across and between various care settings. <u>Examples of some critical questions to ask:</u> A. Does the health care organization, its team leaders and members promote use of adaptive aids to improve mobility, prevent contractures, pressure sores or sensory impairment? - *Are these adaptive aids current or state-of-the-art technology?*
8. Core Knowledge: Ethics	<u>Goals</u>: Assist older adults, families, and caregivers to understand and balance everyday autonomy and safety decisions; apply legal and ethical principles to the complex issues that arise in care of older adults. <u>Examples of some critical questions to ask:</u> A. Do team members actively plan care that includes activities to maintain autonomy and independence in daily living? B. What are the provisions at the health care organization to identify and discuss complex issues that arise with regard to

(Continued)

	Application of AACN's Geriatric Competencies to Assist in Effective Team Building in Long-Term Care *(Continued)*
2.3	

AACN Competency:	Goals and critical questions to ask:
8. Core Knowledge: Ethics (Continued)	autonomous decision making and safety for the older adult resident?
9. Core Knowledge: Human Diversity	<u>Goals</u>: Appreciate the influence of attitudes, roles, language, culture, race, religion, gender, and lifestyle on how families and assistive personnel provide long-term care to older adults. <u>Examples of some critical questions to ask</u>: A. Does the health care organization and its team leaders recognize human diversity among its older adult residents? If so, how is this demonstrated?
10. Core Knowledge: Global Health Care	<u>Goals</u>: Evaluate differing international models of geriatric care. <u>Examples of some critical questions to ask</u>: A. Does the health care organization actively promote transfer of care for older adults from long-term care settings to community dwelling settings if appropriate? B. Have facility policy guidelines been developed that promote early recognition of older adults who could be transitioned to less dependent situations?
11. Core Knowledge: Health Care Systems and Policy	<u>Goals</u>: Analyze the impact of an aging society on the nation's health care system; evaluate the influence of payer systems on access, availability, and affordability of health care. <u>Examples of some critical questions to ask</u>: A. Are the current health care services affordable, accessible, and available to older adults?

(Continued)

	Application of AACN's Geriatric Competencies to Assist in Effective Team Building in Long-Term Care *(Continued)*
2.3	

AACN Competency:	Goals and critical questions to ask:
11. Core Knowledge: Health Care Systems and Policy (Continued)	*Are team members knowledgeable of such services?*
12. Core Knowledge: Provider of Care	Goals: Recognize the benefits of interdisciplinary teams in care of older adults; evaluate the utility of complementary and integrative health practice on health promotion and symptom management Examples of some critical questions to ask: A. Does the facility incorporate use of interdisciplinary teams to carry out clinical care? *Are teams available for consultation purposes?*
13. Core Knowledge: Designer/Manager and Coordinator of Care	Goals: Facilitate older adults' active participation in all aspects of their own health care; involve, educate, and include significant others in implementing best practices for older adults; ensure quality of care commensurate with older adults' vulnerability and frequency/intensity of care needs. Examples of some critical questions to ask: A. Does the team formerly assess or evaluate the older adults' readiness to learn? or their ability to assimilate new information into their plan of care?
14. Core Knowledge: Member of a Profession	Goals: Promote quality preventive and end-of-life care for older adults as essential, desirable, and integral components of nursing practice.

(Continued)

2.3 Application of AACN's Geriatric Competencies to Assist in Effective Team Building in Long-term Care *(Continued)*	
AACN Competency:	**Goals and critical questions to ask:**
14. Core Knowledge: Member of a Profession (Continued)	<u>Examples of some critical questions to ask:</u> A. Does the health care organization and team leaders promote an atmosphere where illness prevention and quality end-of-life care is provided?

Note: Table developed by D. Gray-Miceli.
Source: American Association of Colleges of Nursing. The John A. Hartford Foundation Institute for Geriatric Nursing. (2000). *Older adults: Recommended baccalaureate competencies and curricular guidelines for geriatric nursing care.* Washington, DC: Author.

Reference

Senn, B., Childress, J. R., & Senn, L. E. (2000). *Leadership, teambuilding and culture change: A guide to organizational and personal effectiveness.* Los Angeles: The Leadership Press.

Team Building

Post-test (circle one)

Please circle the *best* answer among the items listed below.

Example:

This is a test.

a. No, this is not a test.
b. Yes, this is a test.
c. No, this is a joke.

The answer is ⓑ so it will be circled.

1. Senn Delaney describe four styles of behavior in their self-scoring behavioral style/instrument. Which style is not described by this inventory?

   a. Controlling
   b. Promoting
   c. Judging
   d. Analyzing

2. There are many characteristics of effective teamwork. What is the major requirement for effective teamwork?

   a. Respect
   b. Openness
   c. Empowerment
   d. Trust

3. A team is

   a. An individual who is working on his/her own to accomplish a goal
   b. A group of people who are independent of each other but work to achieve a common group goal.
   c. A group of people who are dependant on one another to achieve a common goal
   d. None of the above

4. When working with someone with a controlling style, all of the following behaviors are effective EXCEPT:

   a. Spend time on the relationship before jumping to the task
   b. Make your presentation stimulating and exciting
   c. Be decisive and self-confident
   d. Let them do most of the talking

5. Describe your behavioral style. (2 points)
6. Identify the strengths and weaknesses of your style. (4 points)

Participant Evaluation Form

Team Building

Please take the necessary time to respond to each item on this evaluation. Your candid and complete responses are important so that we may improve these educational activities to better meet your learning needs. Thank you.

Module Evaluation

Circle the number that indicates your level of agreement on this form.

A. Objectives:

By the end of this module the learner will be able to:

	Strongly Disagree				Strongly Agree
1. Describe your typical behaviors as a team member using the behavioral inventory assessment tool (Senn-Delaney, 2000).	1	2	3	4	5
2. Discuss the importance of understanding the strengths and weaknesses of different behavioral styles to improve team effectiveness.	1	2	3	4	5
3. Develop a plan to capitalize on one's strengths.	1	2	3	4	5
4. Create a plan to address one's developmental needs.	1	2	3	4	5

B. Overall Purpose:

The purpose of this module is to identify the characteristics of most successful teams and to learn how to achieve these within a team of your choice.

5. Do the above objectives of this module relate to the overall purpose of the program?	1	2	3	4	5

C. Facilities:

The physical facilities were conducive to learning.	1	2	3	4	5

D. Faculty/Teaching Methods:

	Speaker _____ [Insert name] (Team Building)						Speaker Comments
	Very Ineffective			Very Effective			
Expertise in topic area	1	2	3	4	5		
Appropriateness of teaching strategies	1	2	3	4	5		
Ability to make points clear	1	2	3	4	5		
Attitude toward learner	1	2	3	4	5		

E. Miscellaneous:

- Are you familiar with the content in this module? If so, where did you learn it?
- What changes, modifications, or improvements would you suggest before subsequent offering of this module?
- Identify specifically what you intend to do in your professional career with what you learned from this module.
- Comments and suggestions for other programs related to leadership.
- Have you ever taken a leadership course in the past? If so, where, and what were the topics and level (undergraduate, graduate, doctoral, continuing education) of material?
- How long ago did you take this course?_____

Directing and Delegation in Long-Term Care

Pre-test (circle one)

Please circle the *best* answer among the items listed below.

Example

This is a test.

   a. No, this is not a test.
   ⓑ Yes, this is a test.
   c. No, this is a joke.

The answer is ⓑ so it will be circled.

1. If you have delegated a task, you have momentarily transferred the responsibility of the task to _____?

   a. The delegatee
   b. All the people on duty
   c. The charge nurse or nursing supervisor
   d. The delegator

2. If someone has delegated a task, _____ hold(s) the accountability of the task.

   a. The delegatee
   b. All the people on duty
   c. The charge nurse or nursing supervisor
   d. The delegator

3. What must the delegator do for a new patient before assigning tasks to the delegatees?

   a. The delegator can assign any task to the delegatee if they are good friends and the delegator has been working with the delegatee for a long time.
   b. The delegator must assess the patient and make sure the task falls within the practice scope of the delegatee.

c.	The delegator can assign any task to the direct care worker as long as the delegator trusts the direct care worker's judgment.
d.	When it is very busy, the RN delegator can ask the charge nurse (LPN) to carry out any nursing task, because the RN cannot be in two places at the same time.

4.	Choose the letter that constitutes the five (5) rights of delegation from the information below:

1.	Right person
2.	Right thinking
3.	Right task
4.	Right circumstance
5.	Right shift
6.	Right supervision
7.	Right nursing home
8.	Right direction

a.	1, 2, 4, 5, and 7
b.	1, 3, 5, 7, and 8
c.	1, 3, 4, 6, and 8
d.	1, 2, 5, 6, and 7

5.	May the RN delegate the initial assessment of a patient with chest pain to an LPN?

a.	Yes, if the LPN has been working in the nursing home for 10 years.
b.	Yes, if the LPN is attending classes to become a registered nurse.
c.	No, because the patient is experiencing chest pain and initial assessment of chest pain must be done by an RN.
d.	Yes, if the LPN has been taking care of the patient longer than any other worker.

6.	The direct care worker is responsible for the initial assessment of the patient needs and must report findings to the RN as soon as possible.

a.	Yes, the direct care worker knows the long-term care resident the best.
b.	No, the RN or LPN who is in charge has the responsibility of the initial assessment of the resident.

c. No, because the patient may be having a chest pain, and initial assessment of chest pain must be done by an RN.

d. Yes, if the direct care worker is certified and attends a community college nursing program.

7. The direct care worker is allowed to make nursing judgments if she has watched an LPN or RN care for another patient with similar experience in the past at the same facility.

a. Yes, because the direct care worker knows what is right for the residents.

b. No, because the RN or LPN is the only professional who can make nursing judgments.

c. No, because the resident may be having a chest pain, and initial assessment of chest pain must be done by an RN.

d. Yes, if the direct care worker has been taking care of the resident for the longest amount of time.

8. Does the RN need to supervise the direct care worker who has been working in the facility for a long time if the RN delegates a new task to that direct care worker ?

a. No, because the direct care worker is usually certified.

b. No, because the RN or charge nurse is responsible for other services for the residents.

c. Yes, the direct care worker must be supervised for all tasks.

d. Yes, the RN or charge nurse must always supervise the direct care worker when delegating a new task that the direct care worker has not done before.

9. In an urgent situation, in addition to assessing the patient, is the RN/LPN required to also assess the skill of the delegatee before delegation?

a. Yes, because the direct care worker must be assessed to ensure competency.

b. No, if the RN heard that the direct care worker is an exceptional performer.

c. No, because there is no time to do such assessment.

d. No, if the direct care worker is certified.

10. As long as the task falls within the job description of the delegatee, the delegator is not accountable for the task.

a. Yes, because the responsibility has been transferred.

b. No, because the delegator will always be accountable even after delegating responsibility.

c. Yes, otherwise the purpose of delegation is defeated.

d. Yes, especially if the delegatee is certified.

11. Conflict should always be avoided because it stops teamwork. (circle true or false)

True   False

12. Principal causes of conflict within organizations include which of the following:

a. Misunderstandings, value and goal differences

b. Age differences

c. Fluctuating leadership

d. Level of education

13. Which of the following is not an appropriate conflict management mode (select one):

a. Competing

b. Collaborating

c. Lying

d. Compromising

e. Avoiding

14. When giving constructive feedback which of the following approaches is wrong (select one):

a. Convey your positive intent.

b. Make broad general statements rather than focus on specifics.

c. State the impact of the behavior or action.

d. Ask the person to respond.

15. List two (2) action steps necessary to move from conflict to collaboration.

a. _____

b. _____

Directing and Delegation in Long-Term Care

Rita K. Adeniran

and Linda A. Carrick

Today's changing health care environment demands creativity and innovation to accomplish the necessary skills and tasks that will ensure that the National Patient Safety Goals (NPSG) for quality patient care as recommended by the Joint Commission for Accreditation of Healthcare Organizations (JCAHO, 2007). Patient care delivery in long-term care (LTC) requires a multiskilled team approach. For each of these important team members to deliver safe, efficient, and effective health care services, effective human resource utilization and collaboration with adherence to legal boundaries for their respective scope of practice is required.

Navigating regulatory, professional, and organizational boundaries can create confusion and concern for RNs regarding their own liability as it relates to what, when, and how practice can be safely delegated.

Registered nurses (RNs) must be able to employ various leadership skills, including effective direction and delegation, to creatively utilize all health care team members to provide optimal care to patients. Navigating regulatory, professional, and organizational boundaries can create confusion and concern for RNs regarding their own liability as it relates to what, when, and how practice can be safely delegated.

Long-Term Care Services

Although LTC is typically concerned with care of adults over age 65, in fact, all age groups receive long-term care services. In 1994, of the 9 million people receiving LTC, 6.5 million (67%) were 65 years or older (Institute of Medicine [IOM], 2001). Long-term care encompasses services that meet minimal personal assistance, such as basic activities of daily living, to total care needs. It includes a variety of services not limited to medical, social, personal, and other supportive and specialized care. The primary focus of LTC is to support clients to maintain optimal level of functioning—a core function of nursing. Registered nurses and LPNs provide leadership and management in most long-term care settings. Wunderlich and Kohler (2001) reported that in 1998, of the more than 1 million caregivers practicing in nursing homes and personal care facilities, 64.5% were nursing assistants, 18.6% LPNs, and only 14.2% were RNs, with physical therapists and social workers accounting for 2.8%. This chapter will focus on understanding and utilizing the principles of effective directing and delegation to provide optimal care. The chapter objectives include:

Wunderlich and Kohler (2001) reported that in 1998, of the more than 1 million caregivers practicing in nursing homes and personal care facilities, 64.5% were nursing assistants, 18.6% LPNs, and only 14.2% were RNs, with physical therapists and social workers accounting for 2.8%.

- Define directing and delegation.
- Identify the factors that challenge the RN in effective delegation.
- Describe the purpose and importance of delegation.
- Describe legal regulations and professional practice code guidelines about delegation.

- Identify barriers to effective delegation.
- Discuss the process and principle of effective delegation.

Importance of Terms

In discussing directing and delegation and the process of delegation, it is important that professional nurses and other members of the health care team familiarize themselves with the definition of some of the frequently used terms. Table 3.1 provides definitions of frequently used terms in delegation.

Directing

Directing is an act of nursing management. It has been referred to as the leading function of nursing management; the process by which nursing personnel accomplish the objectives of nursing (Marquis & Huston, 2006; Swansburg & Swansburg, 2002). The directing process includes human resource responsibilities, such as motivating, facilitating collaboration, coordinating, delegating, and effectively managing conflict (Marquis & Huston, 2006). Delegating is a major element of the directing process of nursing management; it is an effective management competency by which nurse managers ensure work objectives and accomplishments through employees (Swansburg and Swansburg, 2002). The nurse director or administrator's management style will determine the type of directing that takes place in that organization. For instance, this could either be democratic or autocratic directing. Effective directors inspire subordinates to contribute to organizational goals by coaching and creating harmony between subordinates' roles and the organizational mission.

> The directing process includes human resource responsibilities, such as motivating, facilitating collaboration, coordinating, delegating, and effectively managing conflict.

Delegation

Delegation is the act of empowering one to act on the behalf of another. Delegation is an important nursing function that facilitates timely patient access to selected health care and nursing activities. It is anticipated that when delegation takes effect within the boundaries established by the National Council of State Boards of Nursing (NCSBN) and the American Nurses Association (ANA)

3.1 Terminology in Delegation

Term	Description or Meaning
Accountability	Accountability is when one is responsible and liable for actions and inactions of self and others.
Assignment	Assignment is the transfer of responsibility and accountability of an activity, work from one individual to another. It can also mean a position, post, duty, or office to which one has been designated.
Critical thinking	Critical thinking is the foundation of the reasoning process that involves the application of knowledge and skills, attitudes and values for the purpose of making the best decision that affects patient care.
Decision	Decision is the outcome or determination arrived at after considering different options.
Delegatee	Delegatee refers to the person taking orders in the delegation process, meaning accepting responsibility and authority for the task to be done.
Delegation	Delegation is the act of empowering one to act on the behalf of another.
Delegator	Delegator is the person making the decision to delegate.
Evaluation	Evaluation is the last and probably the most important step of the nursing process. This is when the outcome intervention is reviewed to determine effectiveness of the assessment and implementation actions.
Judgment	Judgment is the formation of an opinion or evaluation by discerning and comparing a formal utterance of an authority's opinion.
Responsible	The responsible person is the individual who is liable to be called on to answer or give explanation for the event or action.
Supervision	Supervision encompasses the critical watching and guiding, directing, and influencing the outcome of an individual performance.
Direct care worker	Direct care worker is any personnel who practices without a license, regardless of title. This individual at most times has been trained to function in an assistive role to the licensed practitioner.

organizational policies, it can improve patient safety and quality of care, while containing the cost of care. In 2006, the NCSBN and the ANA issued a joint statement on nursing delegation (NCSBN, 2006) to emphasize that "all decisions related to delegation are based on the fundamental principles of protection of the health, safety and welfare of the public" (p. 1). Accordingly, most states authorize RNs to delegate as defined within the state practice act. Delegation is a critical skill that may be essential to ensure safe and effective care in an arena of staff shortages, technological advances, and changing infrastructures of care, particularly as hospitals transfer patients with greater acuity of care needs to long-term care services (NCSBN, 2006). According to the ANA (2005), delegation is the "transfer of responsibility for the performance of a task from one individual to another while retaining accountability for the outcome" (p. 4).

The RN Challenge to Effective Delegation

Delegation is a necessity in today's health care environment where resources are scarce. Some evidence suggests that delegation of patient care activities challenges the average RN, specifically those who practice in the long-term settings. According to Parsons (1999), RNs are challenged in particular because they were never taught delegation skills in basic preparation programs at any level. In addition, within the nursing team, there are areas of shared competencies and overlapping roles further complicating delegation to members of the health care team. Moreover, RNs in long-term care are challenged in regards to delegation as scope of practice evolves for health care professionals and because a lack of consistency in organizational and regulatory policies exists across different levels of the care continuum.

In examining characteristics of settings where delegation occurs, nurses may be more likely to delegate in long-term care than acute care (Blegen, Gardner, & McCloskey, 1992). Also, the U.S. Department of Health and Human Services and ASPE (2003) reported to Congress that

> After 2010, the demand for direct care workers in long-term care settings becomes even greater as the baby boomers reach age 85, beginning in 2030 . . . This increase in demand will be occurring at a time when the supply of workers who have traditionally filled these jobs is expected to increase only slightly. (p. v)

Factors that challenge or prevent registered nurses from delegating effectively present the need for ongoing educational efforts and continuing education on ways to effectively manage teams toward quality care. In long-term care, registered nurses direct care of residents with licensed practical nurses (LPNs), licensed vocational nurses (LVNs), and direct care workers. Direct care workers are critical to the provision of care that is individualized and focused on optimal function. One of the challenges in long-term care is the best way to recognize and value the direct care worker. Titles for direct care workers may include nursing assistants (some certified), nursing aides, and in some venues, unlicensed assistive personnel, although this term may evoke a negative response because it emphasizes the lack of a license. In this chapter, we will use the term *direct care worker* to include all of these categories of individuals who provide care under the direction of an RN.

> Direct care workers are critical to the provision of care that is individualized and focused on optimal function.

Parsons (1998), in her research, identified that RNs who attended a structured teaching class about delegation were more satisfied with their jobs. In LTC, job satisfaction is an important component of the health care organization given the high rates of staff turnover and attrition. High turnover, vacancy rates, and difficulty recruiting and retaining skilled nursing professionals are reported across the spectrum of long-term service providers (Castle & Engberg, 2006).

> In LTC, job satisfaction is an important component of the health care organization given the high rates of staff turnover and attrition. High turnover, vacancy rates, and difficulty recruiting and retaining skilled nursing professionals are reported across the spectrum of long-term service providers.

Legal Regulations, Professional Guidelines, and Codes About Delegation

Nursing practice is governed by regulatory, professional, and organizational guidelines as well as codes of ethical conduct. Nurses must delegate functions of care within the boundaries set by these standards. While delegation is not a new strategy that can be used to expand access to selected nursing services, it has become a skill that is critical to effective nursing practice due to constraints of resources and shortage of registered and licensed nurses in long-term care. Most state Nurse Practice Acts (NPA) specifically provide guide-lines for the process of assignment, delegation, and supervision, as well as the legal restrictions for delegation; but no single model of the NPA exists within the United States. Each state defines their own NPA, hence, RNs must practice within the boundaries set by the NPA in their respective state of practice. It is the responsibil-ity of the professional nurse to be knowledgeable of the NPA in their state of practice because variations exist among states in the guidelines for delegation. Lack of awareness of the practice act is not an excuse and cannot serve as a defense. Some Boards of Nursing are empowered to pass rules and regulations that provide specific details not contained in the NPA, about the task and the level that both licensed practitioners and direct care workers can perform.

When directing or delegating, the ANA Code of Ethics for Nurses and its interpretative statements (ANA, 2001) provides guidance for nursing conduct that is consistent with the ethical obligations of the profession as well as high quality nursing care. The Code of Ethics for Nurses informs both the nurse and the public of the profession's expectations and requirements in ethical matters. A code of ethical conduct offers general principles to guide and evalu-ate nursing action. It is important to note that the Code for Nurses is not open to negotiation in employment settings, and the requirements of the Code may often exceed that of the law. Some states have incorporated the ANA Code for Nurses, in part or in total, into state NPAs, thus the nurse has both an ethical and a legal obligation to report certain types of conduct (ANA, 2001).

> It is important to note that the Code for Nurses is not open to negotiation in employment settings, and the requirements of the Code may often exceed that of the law. Some states have incorporated the ANA Code for Nurses, in part or in total, into state NPAs, thus the nurse has both an ethical and a legal obligation to report certain types of conduct.

Some specific codes for nurses that are relevant when direct-ing or delegating from the ANA's Code of Ethics for Nurses (ANA, 2001) include:

- "strives to protect the health, safety, and rights of the pa-tient" (p. 4)
- "responsible and accountable for individual nursing prac-tice and determines the appropriate delegation of tasks consistent with the nurse's obligation to provide optimum patient care" (p. 4)

Section 4.4 of the ANA Code of Ethics for Nurses (ANA, 2001) stipulates that: "the nurse must make reasonable efforts to assess individual competence when assigning selected components of nursing care to other health care workers"(ANA, 2001, p. 17). Therefore, the nurse should not delegate to any member of the nursing team a function for which that person is not prepared or qualified. Employer policies or directives do not relieve the nurse of accountability for making judgments about the delegation of nursing care activities. The complexity of the delivery of nursing care is such that only professional nurses with appropriate education and experience can provide nursing care. Upon employment with a health care facility, the nurse contracts or enters into an agreement with that facility to provide nursing services in a collaborative practice environment. The ANA also outlines nursing care standards that serve to guide nursing practice. For example, the ANA suggests nurses consider these factors in determining appropriate utilization of direct care workers:

"The nurse must make reasonable efforts to assess individual competence when assigning selected components of nursing care to other health care workers" (ANA Code. Section 4.4. p. 17).

- Assessment of the patient condition
- The capability of the direct care worker
- The complexity of the task to be delegated
- The amount of supervision needed and amount the RN will be able to provide
- Number of staff available and workload.

What RNs Can or Cannot Delegate

Registered nurses can only delegate health-related activities that do not require professional nursing skill or judgment. The nurse cannot delegate activities or tasks outside the scope of practice of another skilled health care team member who is not a registered nurse. See Table 3.2 for some functions that can and cannot be delegated to direct care workers.

Risk Associated With Delegation

The RN who delegates still assumes primary responsibility for the patient. Malpractice may occur if the RN inappropriately delegates

3.2 Examples of TASKS That May or May not Be Delegated to the LPNs and Direct Care Workers	
Task That May Be Delegated to the Direct Care Workers	**Task That CANNOT Be Delegated to Direct Care Workers**
❖ Basic personal care duties such as: bathing, grooming, mouth care, comfort measures positioning, making unoccupied bed, and feeding patients ❖ Basic informational gathering such as vital signs and daily weights ❖ Collect, measure, record, and report specific intake and output ❖ Other related activities such as: equipment cleaning and storage, stocking of and restocking of unit supplies, removal of meal trays	❖ Initial nursing assessment of the patient ❖ Assessment requiring professional nursing knowledge, judgment, and professional nurse competencies ❖ Nursing intervention requiring professional nursing knowledge and judgment ❖ Already delegated task ❖ Task requiring the formulation of nursing diagnosis and development of a nursing care plan ❖ Administering medications ❖ Providing patient education

an activity to a direct care worker and does not supervise the direct care worker appropriately. The RN or direct care worker employer and Board of Nursing are responsible for taking disciplinary action against any identified negligence.

The Process and Principles of Effective Delegation

Any step in the process of delegation must take into account the fundamental principle of protecting health, ensuring safety, and providing quality health care for all persons who received nursing care. The authority for the practice of nursing is based on a social contract that acknowledges the professional rights and responsibilities, as well as the mechanism for public accountability (ANA, 2003). Barter (2002) reported that delegation is both an art and a science, involving cognitive, affective, and intuitive dimensions.

Barter maintains that leaders who delegate effectively synchronize the cognitive, affective, and intuitive dimension into a seamless performance. Although delegation is often discussed in isolation or just as a management skill, delegation is actually an integral part of the nursing process that provides an effective framework for how nurses can effectively delegate.

The Nursing Process

Assessment

Barter (2002) notes that assessment of the patient's condition allows the registered nurse to examine and understand the needs of the patient and determine possible outcomes of interventions. Assessment by the nurse will illuminate the complexity of the patient care needs, including the dynamics of the patient status, the acuity level, the technology needed, risk for infection, and the patient's psychological needs. This assessment will also help identify which other health professionals need to be involved in the patient's care and the degree of supervision needed for activities that may be delegated, as well as other environmental factors, such as patient location. Following the nursing assessment, the RN can then identify the component of care that the direct care worker is competent and capable of performing prior to delegating the care. Accurate assessment of the patient condition, as well as the knowledge and competence of the direct care worker, is key to determine whether the task can be safely delegated. See Table 3.2 for information regarding tasks that can be assigned to direct care workers.

> Assessment by the nurse will illuminate the complexity of the patient care needs, including the dynamics of the patient status, the acuity level, the technology needed, risk for infection, and the patient's psychological needs. This assessment will also help identify which other health professionals need to be involved in the patient's care and the degree of supervision needed for activities that may be delegated, as well as other environmental factors, such as patient location.

Planning

The next step in the nursing process of effective delegation is the planning phase. The RN is responsible for the development of the plan of care. Understanding the desirable goal for the client can assist the RN in prioritizing tasks that will be delegated and

ensuring that patients receive optimal care. The RN must understand roles and responsibilities using the five rights of delegation
as stipulated by the NCSBN (1995). The five rights of delegation
can serve as a tool to guide nurses in effectively planning and delegating appropriately. They are:

- The right task
- The right circumstances
- The right person
- The right direction/communication
- The right supervision

After assigning the task to the direct care worker, the RN should
also instruct the direct care worker to call for support if they are
uncertain or unsure about any aspect of care. The direct care
worker must feel assured that bringing uncertainty to a supervisor
or raising questions and asking for help is acceptable and without
threat of reprisal by supervisors or coworkers.

Implementation

For effective implementation of assigned tasks to occur, the direct
care worker must have specific information and a formal assignment to guide them in the delegated task. Registered nurses must
describe the particular task in detail. See Table 3.3 for positive
strategies to implement delegation. Utilizing the four Cs of communication can help to ensure that the direct care worker accurately understands the intervention/implementation task:

Clear:	Does the direct care worker understand what needs to be done?
Concise:	Does the direct care worker have enough information to perform the task?
Correct:	Is the task within the direct care worker's scope of practice? If yes, is the direct care worker competent?
Complete:	What is the desired outcome? Are times and param-eters clear?

This is the last stage and a vital aspect of the delegation process.
It is an ongoing process requiring the RN to provide and obtain

| 3.3 | Positive Power Strategies to Facilitate Effective Delegation |

- Positive self image
- Careful grooming
- Appropriate speech
- Recognizes individual contributions
- Accepts constructive criticism
- Assertive verbal and nonverbal language
- Honesty
- Courteousness
- Friendliness
- Responsibility
- Risk-taking

- Acceptance of wins/losses gracefully
- Ensures that the task meets the legal scope of practice as determined by the State Board of Nursing in the state where the delegation is taking place
- The task should be part of the job description of the organization
- The task must fall within the education of the worker

- The task must meet the policy and procedure description of the organization
- The delegatee must be under the supervision of the delegator as stipulated by the organizational chart.
- The delegatee must be competent and comfortable in performing the task to be delegated

feedback from the direct care workers. Efficiency can be measured if the direct care worker was able to successfully complete the task as delegated, and effectiveness can be measured if the patient reached the defined goal of care. Other considerations for effectiveness are the time frame used by the direct care worker to complete the task and whether the direct care worker accurately reported findings during the task and upon completion of the task. The evaluation process provides an opportunity for the RN to monitor the outcome for delegated tasks and provide feedback to the direct care worker. Discussing the outcome of the delegated task in a safe environment free from reprisals and focused on quality of care with the direct care worker will encourage the direct care worker to ask questions. According to Tappen (1995), supervision and feedback can improve self-confidence.

Guidelines for Effective Delegation

The ANA and NCSBN (2005) joint statements of effective delegation can further provide guidelines to RNs. These are:

- The RN takes responsibility and accountability for the provision of nursing practice.
- The RN directs care and determines the appropriate utilization of any assistant involved in providing direct patient care.
- The RN may delegate components of care but does not delegate the nursing process itself. The practice functions of assessment, planning, evaluation, and nursing judgment cannot be delegated.
- The decision of whether or not to delegate or assign is based upon the RN's judgment concerning the condition of the patient, the competence of all members of the nursing team, and the degree of supervision that will be required of the RN if a task is delegated.
- The RN delegates only those tasks for which they believe the other health care worker has the knowledge and skill to perform, taking into consideration training, cultural competence, experience, and facility policies and procedures.
- The RN individualizes communication regarding the delegation to the nursing assistive personnel and client situation, and the communication should be clear, concise, correct, and complete. The RN verifies comprehension with the nursing assistive personnel and that the assistant accepts the delegation and the responsibility that accompanies it.
- Communication must be a two-way process. Nursing assistive personnel should have the opportunity to ask questions and request clarification of expectations.
- The RN uses critical thinking and professional judgment when following the five rights of delegation outlined previously.
- Directors of Nursing in long-term care are accountable for establishing systems to assess, monitor, verify, and communicate ongoing competence requirements in areas related to delegation.

Barriers to Effective Delegation

Some barriers to delegation include a perceived lack of time, lack of confidence in direct care workers, insecurity of the RN, and fear of ridicule from direct care workers.

Delegation takes time, and it is easy for RNs to believe that it is safer and quicker to do the task alone, even when overwhelmed by other responsibilities. This may undermine trust by team members.

Delegation takes time, and it is easy for RNs to believe that it is safer and quicker to do the task alone, even when overwhelmed by other responsibilities. This may undermine trust by team members. Registered nurses may be unaware of the clinical competencies of the direct care worker and their legal power to use delegation for safe care. They may avoid the responsibilities of delegation and supervision in an effort to be liked by all team members. This can undermine the RNs ability to focus on the more critical care needs of the patients and interfere with earning the respect of the full team as well as persons and families under the care of the RN.

Conclusion

Meeting current health care challenges and benchmarks for quality, cost, and efficiency in long-term care requires effective use of teams. Table 3.4 provides a guide to incorporate geriatric care guidelines when using delegation. Delegating to licensed personnel and direct care workers to carry out selected nursing tasks has been one of the ways that health care facilities, specifically long-term care facilities, have been able to meet the increasing need for accessible, affordable, quality health care services. Delegation is an indispensable skill for professional nursing practice. For nursing to continue to play a key leadership role in long-term care, it is essential that we develop health care teams that work together to provide optimal patient outcomes.

3.4	Application of AACN's Geriatric Competencies in Relation to Directing and Delegation in Long-Term Care
AACN Competency:	Goals and critical questions to ask:
1. Critical Thinking	<u>Goals</u>: Recognize one's own and other's attitudes, values, and expectations about aging and their impact on care of older adults and their families; adopt the concept of individualized care as the standard of practice with older adults.

(Continued)

AACN Competency:	Goals and critical questions to ask:
1. Critical Thinking (Continued)	<u>Examples of some critical questions to ask:</u> A. What are your own, the providers' and team members' style of directing? B. Do the health care organization and team leaders support delegation of nursing activities? C. Does use of delegation in the workplace allow for the provision of individualized care for older adults?
2. Communication	<u>Goals:</u> Communicate effectively, respectfully, and compassionately with older adults and their families; recognize the biopsychosocial, functional, and spiritual changes of old age. <u>Examples of some critical questions to ask:</u> A. Is the health care organization, its staff and team leaders sensitive, knowledgeable and skilled in directing and delegation of activities? If delegation is used within the team approach, is individual competency for selected delegated tasks assessed? Monitored? What are the channels of communication between staff and team members?
3. Assessment	<u>Goals:</u> Incorporate into daily practice valid and reliable tools to assess the biopsychosocial, functional, and spiritual status of older adults; assess the living environment with special awareness of the biopsychosocial and functional changes common in old age; analyze the effectiveness of community resources in assisting older adults and their families to maintain independence; assess family knowledge of skills necessary to deliver care to older adult. <u>Examples of some critical questions to ask:</u> A. Do health care organizations, their team leaders and members delegate unlicensed staff to use assessment tools in the physical assessment process (for routine assessment or for acute emergencies)? Are unlicensed

AACN Competency:	Goals and critical questions to ask:
3. Assessment (Continued)	personnel supervised in this process? Monitored? Or educated about use of such tools? How are older residents safeguarded from inappropriate use of assessment tools? B. Do team leaders and/or team members and staff encourage unlicensed personnel to perform activities beyond an acceptable scope of practice?
4. Technical Skill	<u>Goals</u>: Adapt technical skills to meet the functional, biopsychosocial, and endurance capabilities of older adults; individualize care and prevent morbidity and mortality associated with the use of physical and chemical restraints in older adults. <u>Examples of some critical questions to ask</u>: A. Are staff capable of performing particular technical skills? B. Does the degree of complexity of the task influence who it is delegated to? C. Is health care for the older adult patient fragmented? Non-comprehensive or not individualized when technical skills are assumed or performed by unlicensed personnel?
5. Core Knowledge: Health Promotion, Risk Reduction, Disease Prevention	<u>Goals</u>: Prevent or reduce common risk factors that contribute to functional decline, impaired quality of life, excess disability in older adults; follow standards of care to recognize and report elder mistreatment; apply evidence-based standards to reduce risk, screen, immunize, and promote healthy lifestyles in older adults. <u>Examples of some critical questions to ask</u>: A. Does the health care organization, its team leader or members utilize delegation in their routine assessment and management of various geriatric conditions? (for example, assessment of type 2 diabetes, elder mistreatment, injury prevention, urinary incontinence and polypharmacy?)

(Continued)

AACN Competency:	Goals and critical questions to ask
6. Core Knowledge: Management	**Goals:** Recognize and manage geriatric syndromes common to older adults; recognize the Illness and Disease complex interaction of acute and chronic co-morbidities common to older adults. Examples of some critical questions to ask: A. Do the team leader and health care providers educate all staff and unlicensed personnel about various presentations and the management of geriatric syndromes among older adults? B. Are team members and unlicensed personnel educated to recognize the excess morbidity and mortality associated with diseases?
7. Core Knowledge: Information and Health Care Technology	**Goals:** Use of technology to enhance older adults' function, independence, and safety; facilitate communication through transitions across and between various care settings. Examples of some critical questions to ask: A. Do the team leader and team members educate unlicensed personnel about the various technologies to improve sensory, communication or functional impairment, such as eyeglasses, use of hearing aids, canes, walkers or use of wheelchair and other adaptive devices?
8. Core Knowledge: Ethics	**Goals:** Assist older adults, families, and caregivers to understand and balance 'everyday' autonomy and safety decisions; apply legal and ethical principles to the complex issues that arise in care of older adults. Examples of some critical questions to ask: A. In the health care organization or community setting, do unlicensed personnel participate in ethics meetings, care plans, and discussions related to the older adults' maintenance of

(Continued)

Application of AACN's Geriatric Competencies in Relation to Directing and Delegation in Long-Term Care *(Continued)*

AACN Competency:	Goals and critical questions to ask
8. Core Knowledge: Ethics (Continued)	autonomous decision making? safety? security or ability to live independently?
9. Core Knowledge: Human Diversity	Goals: Appreciate the influence of attitudes, roles, language, culture, race, religion, gender, and lifestyle on how families and assistive personnel provide long-term care to older adults. Examples of some critical questions to ask: A. Do all team members including unlicensed personnel appreciate each and every older adult's diversity?
10. Core Knowledge: Global Health Care	Goals: Evaluate differing international models of geriatric care. Examples of some critical questions to ask: A. What types of health care models have older adult residents experienced from various countries and cultures? How are these acknowledged by health care providers? How are differences addressed or managed?
11. Core Knowledge: Health Care Systems and Policy	Goals: Analyze the impact of an aging society on the nation's health care system; evaluate the influence of payer systems on access, availability and affordability of health care. Examples of some critical questions to ask: A. Are the health care services available to the older adult provided by teams, individual health care providers, or family caregivers?
12. Core Knowledge: Provider of Care	Goals: Recognize the benefits of interdisciplinary teams in care of older adults; evaluate the utility of complementary and integrative health practice on health promotion and symptom management.

(Continued)

	Application of AACN's Geriatric Competencies in Relation to Directing and Delegation in Long-Term Care *(Continued)*
3.4	

AACN Competency:	Goals and critical questions to ask
12. Core Knowledge: Provider of Care (Continued)	<u>Examples of some critical questions to ask:</u> A. Do the health care organization, team leaders, and health care providers recognize, utilize, or explore use of complementary and integrative health care practices when caring for older adults?
13. Core Knowledge: Designer/Manager and Coordinator of Care	<u>Goals:</u> Facilitate older adults' active participation in all aspects of their own health care; involve, educate and include significant others in implementing best practices for older adults; ensure quality of care commensurate with older adults' vulnerability and frequency/intensity of care needs. <u>Critical questions to ask:</u> A. What role do various team members assume in providing health care to older adults? Do unlicensed personnel participate in the education of patients or family caregivers? B. Do unlicensed personnel assist in the identification of frail, vulnerable, or at risk older adult populations?
14. Core Knowledge: Member of a Profession	<u>Goals:</u> Promote quality preventive and end-of-life care for older adults as essential, desirable, and integral components of nursing practice. <u>Critical questions to ask:</u> A. Do team members and unlicensed personnel promote quality preventive and end-of-life care for older adult patients?

Note: Table developed by D. Gray-Miceli.

Source: American Association of Colleges of Nursing. The John A. Hartford Foundation Institute for Geriatric Nursing. (2000). *Older adults: Recommended baccalaureate competencies and curricular guidelines for geriatric nursing care.* Washington, DC: Author.

References

American Nurses Association (ANA). (2001). *Code of ethics for nurses with interpretive statements*. Washington, DC: American Nurses Publishing.

American Nurses Association (ANA). (2003). *Nursing scope and standards of practice*. Washington, DC: American Nurses Publishing.

American Nurses Association (ANA). (2005). *Principles for delegation*. Silver Spring, MD: Author.

American Nurses Association (ANA) and the National Council of State Boards of Nursing (NCSBN). (2005). *Joint statement on delegation*. Retrieved August 18, 2007, from https://www.ncsbn.org/Joint_state ment.pdf

Barter, M. (2002). Follow the team leader. *Nursing Management, 33*(10), 54–57.

Blegen, M. A., Gardner, D. L., & McCloskey, J. C. (1992). Survey results: Who helps you with your work? *American Journal of Nursing, 92*(1), 26–31.

Castle, N. G., & Engberg, J. (2006). Organizational characteristics associated with staff turnover in nursing homes. *The Gerontologist, 46,* 62–73.

Joint Commission on Accreditation of Healthcare Organizations (JCAHO). (2007, September). *National patient safety goals*. Retrieved January 19, 2008 from http://www.jointcommission.org/Patient Safety/NationalPatientSafetyGoals

Institute of Medicine. (2001). *Improving the quality of long-term care*. Washington, DC: National Academy Press.

Marquis, B. L., & Huston, C. J. (2006). *Leadership roles and management functions in nursing: Theory and application* (5th ed.). Philadelphia, PA: Lippincott Williams & Wilkins.

National Council of State Boards of Nursing. (1995). *Delegating concept and decision making process*. National council position paper. Chicago: Author.

National Council of State Boards of Nursing. (2006). *NCSBN and ANA Joint Statement on Nursing Delegation*. Chicago: Author. Retrieved January 21, 2008, from https://www.ncsbn.org/1056.htm

Parsons, L.C. (1998). Delegation skills and nurse job satisfaction. *Nursing Economics, 16*(1), 18–26.

Parsons, L.C. (1999). Building RN confidence for delegation decision making skills in practice. *Journal for Nurses In Staff Development, 6*(15), 263–269.

Swansburg, R.C., & Swansburg, R.J. (2002). *Introduction to management and leadership for nurse managers* (3rd ed.). Sudbury, MA: Jones and Bartlett.

Tappen, R. M. (1995). *Nursing leadership and management: Concepts and practice* (4th ed.). Philadelphia: F. A. Davis.

U.S. Department of Health and Human Services and ASPE. (2003, May 14). *The future supply of long-term care workers in relation to the aging baby boom generation.* Report to Congress. Retrieved August 18, 2007, from http://www.pascenter.org/publications/publication_home.php?id=61

Wunderlich, G. S., & Kohler, P. O. (Eds.). (2001). *Improving the quality of long-term care.* Washington, DC: National Academy Press.

Directing and Delegation in Long-Term Care

Post-test (circle one)

Please circle the *best* answer among the items listed below.

Example

This is a test.

a. No, this is not a test.
(b.) Yes, this is a test.
c. No, this is a joke.

The answer is ⓑ so it will be circled.

1. If you have delegated a task, you have momentarily transferred the responsibility of the task to _____?

    a. The delegatee
    b. All the people on duty
    c. The charge nurse or nursing supervisor
    d. The delegator

2. If someone has delegated a task, _____ hold(s) the accountability of the task.

    a. The delegatee
    b. All the people on duty
    c. The charge nurse or nursing supervisor
    d. The delegator

3. What must the delegator do for a new patient before assigning tasks to the delegatees?

    a. The delegator can assign any task to the delegatee if they are good friends and the delegator has been working with the delegatee for a long time.
    b. The delegator must assess the patient and make sure the task falls within the practice scope of the delegatee.

c. The delegator can assign any task to the direct care worker as long as the delegator trusts the direct care worker's judgment.

d. When it is very busy, the RN delegator can ask the charge nurse (LPN) to carry out any nursing task, because the RN cannot be in two places at the same time.

4. Choose the letter that constitutes the five (5) rights of delegation from the information below:

1. Right person
2. Right thinking
3. Right task
4. Right circumstance
5. Right shift
6. Right supervision
7. Right nursing home
8. Right direction

a. 1, 2, 4, 5, and 7
b. 1, 3, 5, 7, and 8
c. 1, 3, 4, 6, and 8
d. 1, 2, 5, 6, and 7

5. May the RN delegate the initial assessment of a patient with chest pain to an LPN?

a. Yes, if the LPN has been working in the nursing home for 10 years.

b. Yes, if the LPN is attending school to become a registered nurse.

c. No, because the patient is experiencing chest pain and initial assessment of chest pain must be done by an RN.

d. Yes, if the LPN has been taking care of the patient longer than any other worker.

6. The direct care worker is responsible for the initial assessment of the patient needs and must report findings to the RN as soon as possible.

a. Yes, the direct care worker knows the long-term care resident the best.

b. No, the RN or LPN who is in charge has the responsibility of the initial assessment of the resident.

c. No, because the patient may be having a chest pain, and initial assessment of chest pain must be done by an RN.

d. Yes, if the direct care worker is certified and attends a community college nursing program.

7. The direct care worker is allowed to make little nursing judgments if she has watched an LPN or RN care for another patient with similar experience in the past at the same facility.

a. Yes, because the direct care worker knows what is right for the residents.

b. No, because the RN and LPN are the only professionals who can make nursing judgments.

c. No, because the patient may be having a chest pain, and initial assessment of chest pain must be done by an RN.

d. Yes, if the direct care worker has been taking care of the resident for the longest amount of time.

8. Does the RN need to supervise the direct care worker who has been working in the facility for a long time, if the RN delegates a new task to that direct care worker?

a. No, because the direct care worker is usually certified.

b. No, because the RN or charge nurse is responsible for other services for the resident.

c. Yes, the direct care worker must be supervised for all tasks.

d. Yes, the RN or charge nurse must always supervise the direct care worker when delegating a new task that the direct care worker has not done before.

9. In an urgent situation, in addition to assessing the patient, the RN/LPN is required to also assess the skill of the delegatee before delegation.

a. Yes, because the direct care worker must be assessed to ensure competency.

b. No, if the RN heard that the direct care worker is an exceptional performer.

c. No, because there is no time to do such assessment.

d. No, if the direct care worker is certified.

10. As long as the task falls within the job description of the delegatee, the delegator is not accountable for the task.

a. Yes, because the responsibility has been transferred.

b. No, because the delegator will always be accountable even after delegating responsibility.

c. Yes, otherwise the purpose of delegation is defeated.

d. Yes, especially if the delegatee is certified.

11. Conflict should always be avoided because it stops teamwork. (circle true or false)

   True   False

12. Principal causes of conflict within organizations include which of the following:

   a. Misunderstandings, value and goal differences

   b. Age differences

   c. Fluctuating leadership.

   d. Level of education

13. Which of the following is not an appropriate conflict management mode (select one):

   a. Competing

   b. Collaborating

   c. Lying

   d. Compromising

   e. Avoiding

14. When giving constructive feedback, which of the following approaches is wrong (select one):

   a. Convey your positive intent.

   b. Make broad general statements rather than focus on specifics.

   c. State the impact of the behavior or action.

   d. Ask the person to respond.

15. List two (2) action steps necessary to move from conflict to collaboration.

   a. _____

   b. _____

Participant Evaluation Form
Directing and Delegation in Long-Term Care

Today's Date ____/____/____   Facility: _____

Please circle the best response.

Example: Strongly Disagree   Disagree   Agree   Strongly Agree
　　　　　　　　　　1　　　　　　　　2　　　　3　　　　　4

At the end of the presentation I can:

1. Discuss the importance of delegating to LPNs and UAPs (Unlicensed Assistance Personnel).

Strongly Disagree   Disagree   Agree   Strongly Agree
　　　1　　　　　　　　　　2　　　　　　　3　　　　　　　4

2. Explain the PA statuary and regulatory provisions for the delegation of nursing tas and UAPs.

Strongly Disagree   Disagree   Agree   Strongly Agree
　　　1　　　　　　　　　　2　　　　　　　3　　　　　　　4

3. Discuss the five rights of delegation.

Strongly Disagree   Disagree   Agree   Strongly Agree
　　　1　　　　　　　　　　2　　　　　　　3　　　　　　　4

4. Guide others in learning or applying the principles of effective delegation in their daily practice.

Strongly Disagree   Disagree   Agree   Strongly Agree
　　　1　　　　　　　　　　2　　　　　　　3　　　　　　　4

5. Identify the personal and organizational benefits and drawbacks related to conflict management.

Strongly Disagree   Disagree   Agree   Strongly Agree
　　　1　　　　　　　　　　2　　　　　　　3　　　　　　　4

6. Analyze one's conflict style using the five modes of managing conflict.

Strongly Disagree	Disagree	Agree	Strongly Agree
1	2	3	4

7. Discuss strategies for moving from conflict to collaboration.

Strongly Disagree	Disagree	Agree	Strongly Agree
1	2	3	4

8. Identify ways to build trust.

Strongly Disagree	Disagree	Agree	Strongly Agree
1	2	3	4

9. This program will help me work better with other staff.

Strongly Disagree	Disagree	Agree	Strongly Agree
1	2	3	4

Overall, I rate:

10. This program

Poor	Fair	Good	Excellent
1	2	3	4

11. The case scenario

Poor	Fair	Good	Excellent
1	2	3	4

12. Speaker 1 _____ [insert name]

Poor	Fair	Good	Excellent
1	2	3	4

13. Speaker 2 _____ [insert name]

Poor	Fair	Good	Excellent
1	2	3	4

14. This program would be better if:

15. What other management and leadership topics would be helpful to you in the future?

Power and Negotiation

Pre-test (circle one)

Please circle the *best* answer among the items listed below.

Example

This is a test.

   a.   No, this is not a test.
   ⓑ   Yes, this is a test.
   c.   No, this is a joke.

The answer is ⓑ so it will be circled.

Power

1. Power is:

   a.   A characteristic that cannot be learned or acquired.
   b.   Viewed by many nurses to be immoral, corrupting, and contradictory to the caring nature of nursing.
   c.   Strongest when it is given to an individual.
   d.   Not influenced by the situation.

2. Nurses may seek out another nurse who possesses expert knowledge about a clinical procedure. This is an example of what type of power?

   a.   Legitimate power
   b.   Referent power
   c.   Reward power
   d.   Expert power

3. Middle power groups may do all of the following EXCEPT:

   a.   Mediate between high and low groups
   b.   Don't take risks in order to keep the favor of high power groups
   c.   Withhold information and control communication
   d.   Get bought out by one or both groups

4. A strategy a nurse can use to develop a powerful image includes:

   a. Use a phrase such as, "We have a problem."
   b. Take responsibility for communication.
   c. Don't be flexible.
   d. Give little feedback to staff.

5. Describe how you plan to use power as an effective strategy in your workplace setting.

Negotiation

1. Negotiation is the art and science of:

   a. Creating agreements between two groups.
   b. Establishing strategic alliances.
   b. Facilitating the participation of others in decisions.
   c. Pretending to be responsive to other's needs.

2. There are three approaches to negotiation, in the soft positional approach, the individual or group _____.

   a. Concede stubborn!··
   b. Commit early; draf
   c. Focus on interests, not positions
   d. Make threats

3. Positions and interests are important to identify in negotiations. The following are interests EXCEPT:

   a. Needs and concerns
   b. Terms and conditions
   c. Fears and aspirations
   d. Underlying motivations

4. In negotiation, one needs to separate the process of *inventing* possible options for agreement from the process of *deciding among* those options. All of the following would be used as you try to *invent* possible options EXCEPT:

   a. Judging
   b. Improving
   c. Generating
   d. Brainstorming

5. Give one example of effective use of negotiation strategies in your workplace setting.

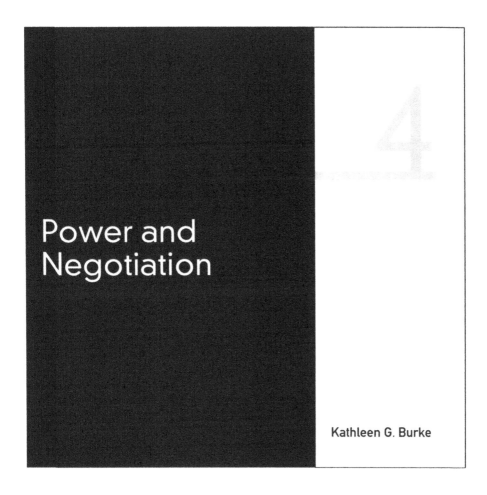

Power and
Negotiation

Kathleen G. Burke

Some people really have almost a distaste for the word [power].
They feel it is alien to conscience. Power for power sake, no. But
the positive use of power for positive purposes is very important. You have to understand that. You've got to have a seat at
the policy table if you want to make a difference.

—*Elizabeth Dole*

The concept of *power* is a complex, elusive, and almost paradoxi-
cal one (Lewicki, Saunders, & Minton, 1999). Effective negotiation
in the health care organization requires an understanding of the
sources of power and how power is used as an effective strategy
in negotiation. In their everyday practice, nurses need and utilize

Effective negotiation in the health care organization requires an understanding of the sources of power and how power is used as an effective strategy in negotiation. In their everyday practice, nurses need and utilize power in order to influence patients, physicians, and other health care professionals.

power in order to influence patients, physicians, and other health care professionals (Manojlovich, 2007). This is an important aspect of nursing leadership that in today's changing health care environment becomes a quintessential aspect of effective health care delivery. As such, nurse leaders need to understand the use(s) of power and how to effectively negotiate agreements so as to continually improve the quality of health care delivered to the older adult in long-term care. Effective use of power transcends all of the 14 core competencies for geriatric nursing care as identified by the American Association of Colleges of Nursing (AACN). In all practice areas, effective use of power is evident through improved communication, assessment, technical skill, and illness and disease management, as well as providing, designing, managing, and coordinating care to older adults.

Purpose

The purpose of this chapter is to examine the major forms and styles of power and negotiation. In this chapter you will become aware of your own power, the power of others, and the negotiation process, and you will learn how to negotiate to be effective leaders in today's health care environment. Further, a critical analysis of this concept is essential to effective strategy negotiations in both one's personal as well as professional life.

By the end of this chapter the learner will be able to:

- Discuss the various types of power,
- Describe the sources of power,
- Describe how to use power as an effective strategy in your workplace environment,
- Discuss the process of negotiation,
- Identify and describe your own negotiation style,
- Describe the effective use of negotiation strategies to achieve personal and professional goals, and
- Utilize power effectively in the workplace to assist in the provision of AACN's essential core competencies for care of the older adult.

Power

Many definitions of *power* have been used in nursing, but for our purposes, power is the ability to influence others to achieve goals (French & Raven, 1960). *Empowerment* is the process by which we facilitate the participation of others in decision making and taking action within an environment where there is equitable distribution of power (Manojlovich, 2007).

Several characteristics exemplify the concept of power. First, it is an acquired characteristic often learned throughout life experiences. Second, use of power is strongest when it is given or acquired by a group. By example, groups tend to accomplish more than single individuals because delegation is often part of the sharing of power. Third, power is influenced by the situational context. People use different types of power depending on the situation. Knowing when and how to use power is an important aspect when one anticipates outcomes such as effective negotiation in the workplace. Sometimes, nurses view power as if it were something immoral, corrupting, or totally contradictory to the *caring* nature of nursing; but the use of power is essential for nurses if they are going to be effective in their roles (Manojlovich, 2007).

> Sometimes, nurses view power as if it were something immoral, corrupting, or totally contradictory to the *caring* nature of nursing; but the use of power is essential for nurses if they are going to be effective in their roles.

Bases of Power

According to French and Raven (1960), there are five common bases of power; these include: *coercive, reward, expert, legitimate,* and *referent.* Each of these bases of power increases a person's capacity to influence the attitudes or behaviors of others. The following section describes each base, or type, of power.

Coercive power is based on fear and the ability to punish. It is use of power in a negative sense to achieve desired outcomes. Fear of being fired from your job, fear of loss in salary, or manipulation of a schedule are examples of how use of coercive power manipulates the work environment. The use of coercive power may get some people to do what you want them to do, but it will not work to influence people for the common goal when fear or the ability to punish is no longer present. A critical thinking point is to identify examples in your work setting where coercive power was used, and then identify how one feels when this type of power is used.

Reward power is the ability to grant awards and favors. It is use of power in a positive sense to achieve desired outcomes. Opposite of coercive power, reward power is a strong motivator to influence people to do things using positive reinforcement. In general, people like to be rewarded with positive comments, favors, gifts, and so forth. This makes people feel good about a job well done or about themselves. Most everyone needs encouragement in daily life. Nurse managers often utilize reward power when they give formal recognition to a staff member who did something special or outstanding for a patient or family member. Recognition of staff who perform their job over and beyond status quo or expectation is a reward for achieving a positive outcome. A critical thinking point is to identify how you may or may not use reward power in your everyday work. How effective do you think giving rewards and favors works with your staff and peers in your ability to influence them? Typically, reward power is very effective if given in appropriate dosages and time intervals. Care must be taken to avoid overuse of reward power.

Reward power is the ability to grant awards and favors. It is use of power in a positive sense to achieve desired outcomes. Opposite of coercive power, reward power is a strong motivator to influence people to do things using positive reinforcement.

Expert power results from utilization of knowledge and skills possessed by an expert that are needed by others. Expert power is based on the perception of someone's competence. Possession of selected information that is needed by others is a form of expert power. Nurses utilize expert power everyday with their patients, families, and with physician providers. Nurses provide care for patients 24 hours a day. Nurses maintain the requisite knowledge as an expert of their patient's health status, response to treatment, and medication. In this sense, nurses maintain expert power because they know foremost the patient's individual needs, strengths, desires, and goals. As such, physician care providers often seek nurses for input on patient care. Nurses are also the most knowledgeable on the standards of care. As described in Table 4.1, nurses can exhibit professional attributes of power in many ways including using business cards, networking for high visibility, or simply taking responsibility for communication with others.

4.1 Professional Attributes

- Belief in value of nursing: Be passionate about your profession and your work. Leaders must have passion for what they do!
- Career commitment/developing expertise: Knowledge is power—ongoing career development is needed for all professional nurses
- Accepting responsibilities
- Taking risks
- Capable of winning and losing gracefully: "Be flexible"
- Be comfortable with conflict and ambiguity
- Give credit when credit is due
- Use constructive criticism not destructive criticism
- Use business cards
- Follow through on promises
- Avoid phrases such as, "We have a problem." Better to say "I have a problem, and I need your help." *Ask for help!*
- Give recognition, praise, thanks, gratitude, and appreciation
- Get the boss's endorsement and support
- Take responsibility for communications
- Networking/high visibility
- Goal setting: Develop 1-year and 5-year goals for yourself
- Organizational savvy: Know your organization's mission; strategic plan and know how your systems work
- Collegiality and collaboration/empowering attitude: Encourage others to accomplish things in your unit
- Developing negotiation skills: Learning how to negotiate will help you to achieve your goals

In units that employ various levels of nursing care, for instance, units with advance practice nurses (APNs), use of expert power is evident. Evidence-based literature supports the use of APNs because they promote positive health care outcomes, improved and coordinated care, and better utlilization of resources (Bourbonnierre & Evans, 2002). As a critical thinking point, can you list some examples of how you use expert power in your everyday work? How effective do you think expert power works with your staff and peers in your ability to influence them? Have you observed that nurses who utilize expert power work collaboratively and cohesively as an effective team compared to situations in which expert power is not utilized?

Legitimate power is based on one's position in an organization or group. Typically, it is associated with having formal job authority or a position of influence on the unit. The nurse manager, nursing supervisor, and nursing director all have legitimate power by virtue of their positions. Registered nurses (RNs) have legitimate power by their formal licenses as RNs. Under ideal circumstances, use of legitimate power by nurses in leadership positions can foster positive outcomes. However, there are also situations to the contrary, where legitimate power can result in adverse outcomes. For example, consider a situation where the unit manager utilizes legitimate power to reframe clinical practice guidelines and how they are utilized on a particular unit. In this case, negative health outcomes can be realized when legitimate power substitutes inappropriately for expert power. A critical thinking point for consideration is: How does your nurse manager use legitimate power on your unit? Can you think of an example where you have used legitimate power as an RN?

> The nurse manager, nursing supervisor, and nursing director all have legitimate power by virtue of their positions. Registered nurses (RNs) have legitimate power by their formal license as RNs. Under ideal circumstances, use of legitimate power by nurses in leadership positions can foster positive outcomes.

Referent power results from followers' desire to identify with a powerful person or power gained by association with people who are perceived as powerful. In any health care organizational system, use of this type of power can be beneficial or detrimental. Nurses frequently use this type of power. Consider these examples: A nurse manger who is liked or admired by his/her staff commands greater follow-through on tasks assigned to subordinate staff than a nurse manager who is not liked. The novice practicing RN admires and may mimic the experienced nurse to achieve positive outcomes in patient care. Besides these examples, can you think of an example on your unit where referent power has been used?

In organizations there are two major kinds of power: position and personal power. Power that a person derives from a position, title, or rank in the formal organization, such as nurse manager, supervisor, or director, is known as *position power*. Position power includes legitimate reward and coercive power. *Personal power* is the influence capacity a person derives from being seen by followers as likable and knowledgeable (Northouse, 2007). For example, some nurses have power because other staff members think of them as good role models. Other nurses have power because the staff thinks of them as highly competent and knowledgeable. Personal power includes referent and expert power (Northouse, 2007).

A case example of the use of different types of power: A head nurse/unit manager has been in charge of the geriatric unit for the past 10 years in a hospital on this subacute, "geriatric step down unit. She is a 'rule oriented person,'" and she makes unilateral decisions with no input from others. She makes all clinical decisions and is the only person who notifies the physician if an emergency arises. As the newly hired RN on the unit, you take a temporary position on the skilled nursing unit until a position opens up for you as the clinical nurse specialist in geriatrics hospital wide. The hospital supervisor asks you to deliver some in-services about geriatric care to that unit to freshen the staff up, and you do so. One day, as you are working as the RN on the unit, several patients develop acute, life-threatening illnesses that are vague in presentation, but obvious to the master's prepared geriatric nurse practitioner (GNP) RN, who is also the only RN on the unit doing assessments. The RN/GNP reports these findings to the head nurse (HN) who discounts their occurrence as unimportant. She calls for monitoring the patient further. One patient has an acute cholecystitis with n/v/d, no fever, and so forth. The Head Nurse argues with the RN and refuses to call the medical doctor (MD). The RN calls the MD anyway (despite policy), and the patient goes to surgery and survives. The MD and surgical staff commend the RN, but the HN gives her a demerit and a write-up saying she went against policy to call the MD. The following week it happens again, but this time, the RN is caring for a 45-year-old woman transferred post-op to the geriatric floor until a bed opens up. The patient has a sudden pulmonary embolism (PE) that is immediately detected by the RN. The RN reports to the HN, but the HN refuses to call the MD, citing not enough clinical evidence. Within 15 minutes of this decision, the patient spikes a 104 fever and has mild wheezing. Soon after, the patient goes into respiratory arrest and dies. There are several issues and types of power related to status and position here: A person in charge with inadequate clinical knowledge in geriatrics and an expert with an underutilized role. The HN used the legitimate power that came with her position as HN to refuse to call the MD, and she used coercive power by giving a demerit and a write up to the RN for calling the physician. The RN used her expert knowledge in recognizing the clinical problem and calling the physician, but in the second example the RN did not use her expert power because she was not empowered to do so by the HN. How do you think this situation could have been handled differently by the HN? And by the RN? How do you manage in a difficult situation like this when the RN's ability to care for their patient is eroded and rendered powerless? How can RNs at the bedside be empowered to provide the best care to their patients? Nurses need to be empowered to use their expert power to provide safe, quality care. Nurses in management positions need to empower their staff to use their expert knowledge and not be tied to rules so that the big picture is lost.

Power Strategies

There are several types of power strategy groups that individuals use in their everyday life and in the workplace. These types of strategies include low power strategies, high power strategies, and mediators. At some point in time, we have all been a member of one or more of these groups. It is important for the nurse to recognize these groups' behaviors so that they can be most effective in influencing groups and individuals toward achievement of a common goal.

Power Groups

Low Power Groups

Individuals in low power groups may demonstrate a number of techniques in an attempt to use power. They may try to use *exposure,* for instance, by "telling others" inside and outside the organization about others' inappropriate behavior. Another example is the threat of chaos: "You keep this up and we will raise havoc here!" Another example is that of moral outrage: "We have justice on our side." Confrontation is sometimes disruptive and sometimes not. Nurses and other health care professionals may engage in these types of behaviors and use of power when they feel out of control of their environment. Analyzing the behavior associated with low power groups can usually identify common patterns.

When nurses in leadership positions recognize these common behaviors and patterns, they may choose to alter previous forms of communication, reporting, and so forth, so as to advert any potential problems created. Channeling negative behavior into positive behavior is therefore an important skill for nurses in practice in leadership positions to acquire.

Channeling negative behavior into positive behavior is therefore an important skill for nurses in practice in leadership positions to acquire.

High Power Groups

People or individuals ascribing to high power groups often use titles, formality, and social distance as a means of achieving power or control of the situation. These groups tend to be highly regulated or rule-oriented and often control who is at the table and the agenda of the group. Some members or leaders ascribing to high power groups may give power away to middle-level or low power groups especially if they feel guilty or awkward about exercising power.

While high power groups are vital to establish and regulate important tasks, the downside is that members may be overcontrolled in the sense that they monopolize or control scarce resources. Characteristic behaviors of members of this high power group range from pretending to challenge and to be responsive while covertly maintaining status quo.

Other recognizable behavior includes use of stalling, or delay (to use up time), while others may withhold information or control communication. Still other behaviors include use of depersonalization and stereotyping low power groups by statements such as "they" aren't like "us." Pattern recognition of these types of behaviors among high power group members can further empower the nurse leader to create counter-strategies.

Middle Power Groups

Middle power groups and individuals don't take risks, so they conserve what power is left or they tend to keep the favor of the high power group. They mediate, or fluctuate, between high and low groups. These groups' members will often insist that the high group "recognize" the low group, or become the low risk groups "friend in court." At times, while waiting for one or both groups to act, group members may become paralyzed. In other instances, ambiguity and insecurity about one's position or role may surface, making decision making challenging. Nurse managers are often in this middle power group.

Strategies for Developing Powerful Image

Given all of the various types of power and ranges of group members' behaviors, nurse leaders must be able not only to recognize the behavior through critical analysis and assessment, but to be poised to do something about it. When management strategies change because of heightened awareness, then effective positive health care outcomes for the organization and the patients served within that organization can be achieved. This requires the nurse to use several strategies to create a powerful image for themselves and their staff.

> When management strategies change because of heightened awareness, then effective positive health care outcomes for the organization and the patients served within that organization can be achieved.

Nurses can use several strategies to create a powerful image for themselves and their staff (see Table 4.2).

Negotiation

Negotiation is the art and science of creating agreements between two parties. Nursing reflects a series of effective, successful negotiations, and effective nurse leaders require successful negotiation. Nurses negotiate with patients to help deliver their care, they negotiate with physicians on how to deliver care, and they negotiate with their peers and with nursing administration. Skills in negotiation are essential in influencing people and facilitating constructive positive relationships in the complex health care environment.

> Negotiation is the art and science of creating agreements between two parties.

Negotiating Process

The negotiating process begins at the so-called *bargaining table.* Each person presents an opening position, and the process moves

4.2 Strategies for Developing a Powerful Image

Personal Attributes	Personal Demeanor	Speech	Style	Overall Behaviors and Mannerisms
Belief in power as a positive force	Be flexible — the health care system is a very complex, fluid environment	Speech: use of voice tone and inflection are important aspects of effective communication to peer staff as well as patients	Grooming and dress	Always be courteous and respectful of staff and patients
Honesty and trust are the most important things needed to build a team	Learn how to deal with change	How individuals perceive and receive the information delivered, verbally and non-verbally, shapes whether or not the communication is received positively or negatively	Wear clean, professional, appropriate attire	Body language/use of touch

(Continued)

4.2 Strategies for Developing a Powerful Image (Continued)

Personal Attributes	Personal Demeanor	Speech	Style	Overall Behaviors and Mannerisms
Create a positive self image through caring for yourself	Don't take things personally; problems are never about you; look for the real issues/concerns	Ideally, clear, positive communication strategies are the gold standard		Smile
Keep a balance between work, family, and social life				
Improve on strengths; don't concentrate on weaknesses				

on until they reach a mutually agreeable result, or until both parties walk away from the unsuccessful process. There are several approaches to negotiation: the soft position, the hard position, and the problem-solving approach. Each approach may be used in a variety of different settings and in different contexts.

There are several approaches to negotiation: the soft position, the hard position, and the problem-solving approach. Each approach may be used in a variety of different settings and in different contexts.

Soft Positional. The use of the soft positional approach includes avoidance of conflict, and the people in the negotiation are viewed as friends. The negotiator tends to change their position easily to avoid a contest of wills and make concessions for the relationship. They may back down to ultimatums and commit early.

Hard Positional. The use of the hard positional approach includes the position that winning is the most important result. The people in the negotiation are adversaries. They dig into their positions, and if they need to concede, they do so stubbornly. In this approach, winning is a contest of will. There is a demand for concessions to have a relationship, they make threats, and commit early.

Problem Solving. In the use of the problem-solving approach, the negotiator attempts to solve the problem; treats parties like professionals; focuses on interests, not positions; and does not concede anything. The negotiator invents options and uses standards of independence of will outside evidence of practice. The negotiator separates the people from the problem and knows each side's best walkway alternative. To reach closure in a problem-solving approach, you draft as you go, and you commit only to a solution at the end. This is a very effective approach to negotiation for the nurse to use with their patients and staff. It uses critical thinking as a strategy for effective problem solving.

Two important things to point out about negotiation are the differences between someone's position and someone's interests. A person's position is the thing they want or demand, that is, their terms and conditions. They are the things the person says they will or won't do. A person's interests are the underlying motivations, needs, concerns, fears, and aspirations. It is important to focus on

A person's interests are the underlying motivations, needs, concerns, fears, and aspirations. It is important to focus on the party's interest and not their position when you are negotiating.

the party's interest and not their position when you are negotiating.

There are two possible approaches in the development of an agreement that can be utilized in a negotiation: inventing or deciding options. When you are *deciding* options, you choose among options and commit to one of those options. In using this option, the negotiator tends to focus on judging, narrowing, arguing, and evaluating the options.

When you are *inventing* options during a negotiation you are not committing, you are looking for improving options, generating new options, brainstorming, and suspending judgment on all options. When you are generating options there is no criticism and no commitment. You are inventing many options so that you can meet the interests of both sides. The negotiator does not evaluate during brainstorming and dovetails differing interest for mutual gain.

In the negotiation process, there are two ways to talk about an issue: (1) talk *at* the other side by focusing on the past, talking about who is right, blaming them for the problem, and trying to score points; or (2) talk *with* the other side by focusing on the future, talking about what is to be done, tackling the problem jointly, clarifying the interests, and inventing new options. This is the more productive way to negotiate in the complex health care environment.

Can you think of a recent example where you needed to negotiate for something for your patient? See Table 4.3 for approaches relevant to geriatric care. What approach did you use? How effective was that approach? Did you know what the party's position and interests were? Did you develop new options? Would you change the way you negotiated?

Conclusion

The purpose of this chapter was to examine the major forms and styles of power and negotiations. In this chapter we discussed the types of power, the power of others, and how to use power and negotiations to effect quality patient care. Power is complex, power is relational, and negotiations skills are essential for nurses. Knowledge really is power, and the use of knowledge to effect change is essential in the complex environment of long-term care.

4.3	Application of AACN's Geriatric Competencies in Relation to Power and Negotiation in Long-Term Care	

AACN Competency:	Goals and critical questions to ask:
1. Critical Thinking	**Goals:** Recognize one's own and others' attitudes, values, and expectations about aging and their impact on care of older adults and their families; adopt the concept of individualized care as the standard of practice with older adults. **Examples of some critical questions to ask:** A. What are your own, the providers', and team members' concepts of power, and how is it used as an effective strategy in the workplace? B. How can power be used to identify attitudes about aging? How can power (for instance reward, expert, legitimate, or referent) be used to influence others' attitudes or behaviors about aging in the workplace? C. Is there sharing of power within the team? How do you know?
2. Communication	**Goals:** Communicate effectively, respectfully, and compassionately with older adults and their families; recognize the biopsychosocial, functional, and spiritual changes of old age. **Examples of some critical questions to ask:** A. Are the health care organization, its staff, and team leaders sensitive, knowledgeable, and skilled in their communication to older adults and their families without use of coercive power or forms of communication?
3. Assessment	**Goals:** Incorporate into daily practice valid and reliable tools to assess the biopsychosocial, functional, and spiritual status of older adults; assess the living environment with special awareness of the biopsychosocial and functional changes common in old age; analyze the effectiveness of community resources in assisting older adults and their families to maintain independence; assess

(Continued)

AACN Competency:	Goals and critical questions to ask:
3. Assessment (Continued)	family knowledge of skills necessary to deliver care to older adults.
	<u>Examples of some critical questions to ask:</u>
	A. Do health care organizations, their team leaders, and members utilize personal or position power to teach about use of assessment tools and techniques for history taking among older adults? B. Are barriers created by team members or their approach (due to use of coercive power) that prohibit effective teaching to family members or patients about their condition and its management? If so, how can this barrier be eliminated?
4. Technical Skill	<u>Goals:</u> Adapt technical skills to meet the functional, biopsychosocial, and endurance capabilities of older adults; individualize care and prevent morbidity and mortality associated with the use of physical and chemical restraints in older adults.
	<u>Examples of some critical questions to ask:</u>
	A. Are staff knowledgeable, and can they be trained on technical skills unique to caring for older adults? *Are staff resistant to change behavior or to adapt technical skills needed to provide quality care to older adults? If so, how can this barrier be effectively managed? What sort of power would you use? What are the steps in the negotiation process for change in this practice?*
5. Core Knowledge: Health Promotion, Risk Reduction, Disease Prevention	<u>Goals:</u> Prevent or reduce common risk factors that contribute to functional decline, impaired quality of life, excess disability in older adults; follow standards of care to recognize and report elder mistreatment; apply evidence-based standards to reduce risk, screen, immunize, and promote healthy lifestyles in older adults.

(Continued)

AACN Competency:	Goals and critical questions to ask:
5. Core Knowledge: Health Promotion, Risk Reduction, Disease Prevention (Continued)	<u>Examples of some critical questions to ask:</u> A. Does the health care organization, its team leader or members utilize established national clinical guidelines for the assessment and management of various conditions unique to care of older adults? (For example, assessment of type 2 diabetes, elder mistreatment, injury prevention, urinary incontinence and polypharmacy?) If not, how do nurse leaders negotiate for such a change in policy and practice?
6. Core Knowledge: Illness and Disease Management	<u>Goals:</u> Recognize and manage geriatric syndromes common to older adults; recognize the complex interaction of acute and chronic comorbidities common to older adults. <u>Examples of some critical questions to ask:</u> A. Does each team member recognize various presentations and the management of geriatric syndromes among older adults? If not, as the nurse leader, what strategies would you negotiate so that health care team members are knowledgeable?
7. Core Knowledge: Information and Health Care Technology	<u>Goals:</u> Use of technology to enhance older adults' function, independence, and safety; facilitate communication through transitions across and between various care settings. <u>Examples of some critical questions to ask:</u> A. Do the team leader and team members recognize the meaning, value, and beliefs held by older adults who utilize various technologies to improve sensory, communication, or functional impairment, such as eyeglasses, use of hearing aids, canes, walkers, or use of wheelchair and other adaptive devices? If not, as team leader, what strategies would you negotiate with upper-level management?

(Continued)

AACN Competency:	Goals and critical questions to ask:
8. Core Knowledge: Ethics	<u>Goals:</u> Assist older adults, families, and caregivers to understand and balance everyday autonomy and safety decisions; apply legal and ethical principles to the complex issues that arise in care of older adults. <u>Examples of some critical questions to ask:</u> A. In the health care organization or community setting, does use of coercive power exist and pose a threat to the older adults' autonomous decision making? Safety? Security or ability to live independently? *If so, as team leader, how would you advocate for the rights of the older adult? What strategies would you employ?*
9. Core Knowledge: Human Diversity	<u>Goals:</u> Appreciate the influence of attitudes, roles, language, culture, race, religion, gender, and lifestyle on how families and assistive personnel provide long-term care to older adults. <u>Examples of some critical questions to ask:</u> A. Does the health care facility take the necessary steps to ensure delivery of quality health care to all residents equally? What guidelines or protocols are used if any?
10. Core Knowledge: Global Health Care	<u>Goals:</u> Evaluate differing international models of geriatric care. <u>Examples of some critical questions to ask:</u> A. Does the facility incorporate state-of-the-science programs and models for delivery of high-quality care to older adults? If not, why not? And, as team leader, what steps could you take to explore these possibilities?
11. Core Knowledge: Health Care Systems and Policy	<u>Goals:</u> Analyze the impact of an aging society on the nation's health care system; evaluate the influence of payer systems on access, availability, and affordability of health care.

(Continued)

AACN Competency:	Goals and critical questions to ask:
11. Core Knowledge: Health Care Systems and Policy (Continued)	Examples of some critical questions to ask: A. Are the health care services available to the older adult utilized? Are they affordable? Accessible? And are they appropriate for older adults? If not, as team leader, how would you negotiate for this change?
12. Core Knowledge: Provider of Care	Goals: Recognize the benefits of interdisciplinary teams in care of older adults; evaluate the utility of complementary and integrative health practice on health promotion and symptom management. Examples of some critical questions to ask: A. Do the health care organization, team leaders, and health care providers recognize, utilize, or explore use of complementary and integrative health care practices when caring for older adults of diverse cultures? If not, why not? What types of power and negotiation strategies would you utilize as team leader and provider of care?
13. Core Knowledge: Designer/Manager and Coordinator of Care	Goals: Facilitate older adults' active participation in all aspects of their own health care; involve, educate, and include significant others in implementing best practices for older adults; ensure quality of care commensurate with older adults' vulnerability and frequency/intensity of care needs. Critical questions to ask: A. Are there barriers influencing the older adults' participation or education about health care activities? If so, as team leader, how can you negotiate for change?

(Continued)

4.3	Application of AACN's Geriatric Competencies in Relation to Power and Negotiation in Long-Term Care *(Continued)*
AACN Competency:	**Goals and critical questions to ask:**
14. Core Knowledge: Member of a Profession	<u>Goals:</u> Promote quality preventive and end-of-life care for older adults as essential, desirable, and integral components of nursing practice. <u>Critical questions to ask:</u> A. Does the health care organization and team members provide quality preventive and end-of-life care for older adults? If not, as team leader, what strategies would you negotiate to ensure that quality patient care occurred?

Note: Table developed by D. Gray-Miceli.

Source: American Association of Colleges of Nursing. The John A. Hartford Foundation Institute for Geriatric Nursing. (2000). *Older adults: Recommended baccalaureate competencies and curricular guidelines for geriatric nursing care.* Washington, DC: Author.

References

Bourbonniere, M., & Evans, L. K. (2002). Advanced practice nursing in the care of frail older adults. *Journal of the American Geriatrics Society, 50,* 2062–2076.

French, J., & Raven, F. (1960). The bases for social power. In C. Cartwright & A. Zander (Eds.), *Group dynamics.* Evanston, IL: Row and Peterson. pp. 607–623.

Lewicki, R. J., Saunders, D. M., & Minton, J. W. (1999). *Negotiation* (3rd ed.). New York: McGraw-Hill.

Manojlovich, M. (2007, January 31). Power and empowerment in nursing: Looking backward to inform the future. *OJIN: The Online Journal of Issues in Nursing, 12*(1), manuscript 1. Retrieved January 24, 2008, from http://www.nursingworld.org/ojin/topic32/tpc32_1.htm

Northouse, P. G. (2007). *Leadership theory and practice* (4th ed.). Thousand Oaks, CA: Sage Publications.

Power and Negotiation

Post-test (circle one)

Please circle the *best* answer among the items listed below.

Example

This is a test.

   a.   No, this is not a test.
   ⓑ   Yes, this is a test.
   c.   No, this is a joke.

The answer is ⓑ so it will be circled.

Power

1. Power is:

   a.   A characteristic that cannot be learned or acquired.
   b.   Viewed by many nurses to be immoral, corrupting, and contradictory to the caring nature of nursing.
   c.   Strongest when it is given to an individual.
   d.   Not influenced by the situation.

2. Nurses may seek out another nurse who possesses expert knowledge about a clinical procedure. This is an example of what type of power?

   a.   Legitimate power
   b.   Referent power
   c.   Reward power
   d.   Expert power

3. Middle power groups may do all of the following EXCEPT:

   a.   Mediate between high and low groups
   b.   Don't take risks in order to keep the favor of high power groups
   c.   Withhold information and control communication
   d.   Get bought out by one or both groups

4. A strategy a nurse can use to develop a powerful image includes:

   a. Use a phrase such as, "We have a problem."
   b. Take responsibility for communication.
   c. Don't be flexible.
   d. Give little feedback to staff.

5. Describe how you plan to use power as an effective strategy in your workplace setting.

Negotiation

1. Negotiation is the art and science of:

   a. Creating agreements between two groups.
   b. Establishing strategic alliances.
   c. Facilitating the participation of others in decisions.
   d. Pretending to be responsive to other's needs.

2. There are three approaches to negotiation, in the soft positional approach, the individual or group _____.

   a. Concede stubbornly
   b. Commit early; draft late
   c. Focus on interests, not positions
   d. Make threats

3. Positions and interests are important to identify in negotiations. The following are interests EXCEPT:

   a. Needs and concerns
   b. Terms and conditions
   c. Fears and aspirations
   d. Underlying motivations

4. In negotiation, one needs to separate the process of *inventing* possible options for agreement from the process of *deciding among* those options. All of the following would be used as you try to *invent* possible options EXCEPT:

   e. Judging
   f. Improving
   g. Generating
   h. Brainstorming

5. Give one example of effective use of negotiation strategies in your workplace setting.

Participant Evaluation Form

Power & Negotiation

Please take the necessary time to respond to each item on this evaluation. Your candid and complete responses are important so that we may improve these educational activities to better meet your learning needs. Thank you.

Module Evaluation

Circle the number that indicates your level of agreement on this form.

A. Objectives:

By the end of this module the learner will be able to:

	Strongly Agree			Strongly Disagree	
1. Discuss the various types of power.	1	2	3	4	5
2. Describe the sources of power.	1	2	3	4	5
3. Describe how to use power as an effective strategy in your workplace environment.	1	2	3	4	5
4. Discuss the process of negotiation.	1	2	3	4	5
5. Describe your own negotiation style.	1	2	3	4	5
6. Describe the effective use of negotiation strategies to achieve personal and professional goals.	1	2	3	4	5

B. Overall Purpose:

The overall purpose of this project is to develop and strengthen RN skills in leadership, management, cultural competency, adult education, and geriatric care excellence in geriatric and long-term care settings

1. Do the objectives of this module relate to the overall purpose of the program?	1	2	3	4	5

93

2. Will the information be useful
   in your professional career?   __ Yes   __ No

Comments:

C. Facilities:

The physical facilities were
conducive to learning.   1   2   3   4   5

D. Faculty/Teaching Methods:

	Speaker _____ [Insert name] (Power and Negotiation)					
	Very Ineffective			Very Effective		Speaker Comments
Expertise in topic area	1	2	3	4	5	
Appropriateness of teaching strategies	1	2	3	4	5	
Ability to make points clear	1	2	3	4	5	
Attitude toward learner	1	2	3	4	5	

E. Miscellaneous:

- Are you familiar with the content in this module? If so, where did you learn it?
- What changes, modifications, or improvements would you suggest before subsequent offering of this module?
- Identify specifically what you intend to do in your professional career with what you learned from this module.
- Comments and suggestions for other programs related to leadership.
- Have you ever taken a leadership course in the past? If so, Where and what were the topics and level (undergraduate, graduate, doctoral, continuing education) of material?
- How long ago did you take this course?_____

Change Theory and Process

Pre-test (circle one)

Please circle T if the statement is True and F if the statement is False.

1. Everyone's initial response to change is anger.

   T   F

2. Two requirements for effective individual change are willingness and anxiety related to potential job loss.

   T   F

3. It is important for a leader to spend energy and time on all employees, especially those most resistant to change.

   T   F

4. Individual responses to change can progress from denial to resistance to exploration and then commitment.

   T   F

5. When individuals are in a resistant mode, it is important for the leader to continue to give them information and direction.

   T   F

6. During times of change, resilience is perceived as a negative attribute.

   T   F

7. To lead change a leader must be passionate, have a vision, and accept stumbles, falls, and move forward.

   T   F

Please circle the item that is not a characteristic.

8. Characteristics of change include all of the following EXCEPT:
   a. Evokes multiple responses
   b. It's inevitable and ever-present
   c. Slow paced and requires consensus
   d. Can be disruptive, intrusive, and upsets status quo

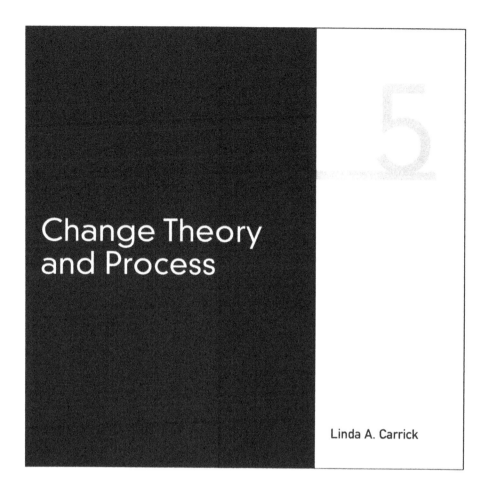

Change Theory and Process

Linda A. Carrick

Change is inevitable; growth is optional. Change is a process of moving from one state or condition to another. Change is not a single event, it is a process. There is planned and unplanned change. In today's health care environment, employees are experiencing tremendous changes in practice, workflow, patient expectations, organizational strategies, and how teams work together.

Utilization of the process of change in practice allows nurses to integrate the American Association of Colleges of Nursing (AACN) core competency in their delivery of quality health care to older adults (AACN, 2000). For example, in order to meet the health care needs of older adults in long-term care, nurse leaders and managers constantly upgrade educational programs and services by integrating the influx of new knowledge and technical skill in each and every patient encounter. This allows for the delivery of state-of-the-science knowledge and evidence-based practice. Without such a change represented by integration of new knowledge into practice, health care becomes outdated and stagnate and can lead to adverse health care outcomes.

In order to understand change as it relates to the health care organization, this chapter will address planned and unplanned change theorists, the processes of change, as well as leading and managing change.

Overview of Change

There are five unique characteristics of change: (1) It is inevitable and ever-present; (2) it is more rapid-paced than ever before; (3) it evokes multiple responses; (4) it offers excitement, opportunity, and challenge; and (5) it can be disruptive and intrusive, and it upsets the status quo (Karp, 1996). Overall, we cannot control change, but we can control our responses to change.

Every individual change effort requires both the ability and the willingness to change to be successful. *Ability* refers to knowledge and skills necessary to adopt the new behavior. *Willingness* refers to attitudes and feelings one holds regarding the required or actual change. Often we assume staff is resisting change when in fact they may not have the ability or preparation necessary to implement the required change. For example, if there is a practice change required, but the staff seem resistant or unwilling to changing their practice, a conflict exists. The first step in resolving this conflict is to explore if the staff has had the education and training necessary to change practice. If not, steps must be taken to increase the staff members' ability to adopt the new behavior, for instance, by the educational process. If staff is observed to have acquired the technical skill following the educational seminar, but they continue to be resistant or unwilling to change their practice, then the conflict may reside with issues related to their willingness to be part of the team. Typically, when one critically analyzes the situation by considering if it is a willingness issue or an ability issue, solutions for change become evident. Let's consider some of the major change theorists and their work.

Ability refers to knowledge and skills necessary to adopt the new behavior. *Willingness* refers to attitudes and feelings one holds regarding the required or actual change.

Change Theories/Theorists

For the past 40 years, change theorists studied types of change, watched people change over time, and followed the leaders of change. Planned change theory dominated the 1950s, '60s and '70s. In planned change theory, there is a deliberate decision made to change. Planned change says that if you follow some modification of the problem-solving process you can implement change and move forward, and you will get from point A to point B. To understand how this is applicable requires knowledge of the problem-solving process. In all, the problem-solving process includes four discrete stages: (1) Define the problem; (2) develop strategies; (3) implement strategies; and (4) evaluate outcomes, and then begin again if necessary. Planned change is deliberate and usually affects a confined group of people. According to this theory, it is recommended to have a change agent. The role of the change agent is to help people change, help them understand change is needed to get by, and help people get comfortable with the change anticipated. Use of a change agent facilitates the process of change.

Initially, change theorists focused on change as a planned process. Kurt Lewin (1951) defined the planned change process as unfreezing, moving, and refreezing. According to Lewin, change occurs based on driving forces and resisting forces and is exemplified when the driving forces exceed the restraining forces (Yoder-Wise, 1999).

> The role of the change agent is to help people change, help them understand change is needed to get by, and help people get comfortable with the change anticipated. Use of a change agent facilitates the process of change.

In 1958, Lippitt, Watson, and Westley expanded the work of Lewin (1951) to five phases of change: (1) unfreezing, (2) creating a change relationship, (3) moving, (4) refreezing, and (5) ending the change contract. Havelock (1973) also expanded these theories to create change by following a seven-step process: (1) build relationships, (2) gain acceptance, (3) diagnose the problem, (4) acquire needed resources, (5) choose a solution, (6) stabilization, and (7) self-renewal (Yoder-Wise, 1999). Planned change is good, but it has to be simple and doesn't require a lot of buy in. In today's health care environment, things are often not simple; therefore an organization may follow this seven-step approach and still not be able to reach sustainable change.

Rogers (1995) is the more contemporary planned change theorist. He defined the process of change as awareness, interest, evaluation, trial, and then adoption of change.

Taking all of the elements combined, planned change constitutes these attributes/characteristics:

- Deliberately engineered with predetermined goals
- Linear process (directional and sequential)
- Occurs in groups, using change agent to lead
- Alters ways of doing things in social systems using problem-solving methods
- Effective for low-level complexity changes

Unplanned Change

Unplanned change is reactive to its environment. For example, I'm watching the environment, and I see an opportunity, and I make a change to follow the vision.

Characteristics of unplanned change include the following:

- Change is a nonlinear process that is reactive to the environment.
- Change is dynamic, responsive, and flexible.
- Change is effective with complex realities.
- Change is based on shared values and vision (you have to be passionate).
- Change places an emphasis on relationships.
- Change requires information and communication.

A well-known unplanned change theorist is Peter Senge (1990). Senge believes in the learning organization, where you have systems thinking, personal mastery, mental models, building shared vision, and team learning. Maybe the most relevant in unplanned change theorist is McDaniel's (1996) chaos theory. McDaniel believes organizations are open systems operating in complex, fast-changing environments with order emerging through fluctuation and chaos, but never the same form. McDaniel states that "healthcare organizations cannot control long term outcomes." The challenge of the leaders in health care is to make sense of the chaos.

The value of change theory is to help us understand. It helps us develop an understanding of what is happening around us; it helps us compare similarities and differences of planned and unplanned change; it helps us

> McDaniel states that "healthcare organizations cannot control long term outcomes." The challenge of the leaders in health care is to make sense of the chaos.

decide whether to respond or lead change; and it helps us assess ways to lead change based on understanding how change occurs (bag of tricks). Realistically in daily life, we often use the concepts of both planned and unplanned change depending on what the desired change entails.

Responses to Change

People react to change in different ways. Examples of responses to change can be positive, negative, or neutral as illustrated by the statement, "What's in it for me?" All in all, one cannot control change, but we can control our response to change. How we respond to change is entirely up to us. We can decide to react positively or negatively to change introduced from external forces. We could also wait for others to tell us what is going on and whether it is safe to change. Another option is to decide to lead change.

When change is implemented individuals can go through four phases, beginning with denial, which can include anger, bargaining, and a sense of loss (Tiffany & Lutjens, 1998). Resistance is the second phase, during which individuals experience confusion and hopelessness. If individuals are capable of moving out of the resistance phase, they can then move into exploration. During exploration individuals are open to a level of acceptance and adjustment. It is in this phase that the leader must reach out and encourage involvement and participation in the change process. The last phase is commitment, during which there is acceptance and a renewed sense of commitment. Moving people through each phase requires active participation from the leader. All people will not move through these phases at the same time. Therefore the leader must develop interventions to move individuals through the stages of change (Tiffany & Lutjens, 1998, Ch. 2).

Change is a process, and everyone goes through the process differently. Transition does not just happen. We all go through the stages of change, but our timelines are different based on our own personal experiences with change. Transformational leaders must create a shared vision that provides direction, motivation, and commitment toward a common goal (Table 5.1). Communication is one of the most important components of change. Not communicating to employees during a major organizational change is a mistake. Communication should include the facts, be done face-to-face, and utilize frontline managers. It is important to communicate values through actions, not words. The leader must "walk the walk and talk the talk." The nurse leader is responsible for establishing and communicating the vision. Usually it's the chief nursing officer who passionately articulates the vision and demonstrates unwavering commitment. The nurse managers and directors must be willing to embrace the vision and effectively communicate the vision and strategies to the staff and other members of the health care team (Marley & Reck, 2006). Mid-level managers have the ability to strongly influence and support the staff during the change process.

Communication is one of the most important components of change.

The role of senior management is to communicate and empower the frontline supervisors with the information needed to promote a positive change. The literature supports that employees would rather receive information from their immediate supervisor than from senior management (Larkin & Larkin, 1996). Communication is perceived as more credible from someone they interact with on a regular basis and may trust.

As mentioned earlier, *ability* and *willingness* are needed for change. Resilience is also an important component. Resilience is the ability to readjust one's expectations to the new reality. Resilient people are able to stay focused, be flexible, remain organized, engage in change, and see change as positive. A positive attitude and resilience are linked (Coutu, 2002). During times of change, it is important to take care of yourself; identify and use tools and techniques to help you transition. Table 5.2 illustrates ways of facilitating change. Overall, there are seven basic strategies that

5.1	Transition Process and What Leaders Should Do
Transition Phase:	**Leaders' Response:**
Denial	Give information and empathize
Resistance	Listen and communicate
Exploration	Encourage and help people focus their energy
Commitment	Validate, reward, celebrate

make change easier for employees and persons in management. Adherence to these principles can help to facilitate the change process (Table 5.2).

In Johnson's book *Who Moved My Cheese?* (1998), he identified animated characters (mice and little people) and their responses to change—someone moved their cheese. This analogy allows us to look at our behavior as it relates to our reaction to change. Do we accept change and move into action, or do we wait and complain about the change and hope that it never occurs? Table 5.3 illustrates some of the reactions of the characters in the book.

5.2 The Seven Interventions to Make the Change Process Easier

1. Take time to understand what the change is about.
2. Think before you react.
3. Recognize what you can take with you to make the transition more comfortable.
4. Explore the positive side of change.
5. Find someone to talk to.
6. Explore what is waiting in the new beginning.
7. Use transitions as an impetus to learn and grow.

5.3 Characters and Their Reactions in *Who Moved My Cheese?* (Johnson, 1998)

Character presented:	Possible reactions:
SNIFF?	Who can smell change in the air?
SCURRY?	Who goes into action immediately?
HEM?	Who does not want to change? "It's not fair"
HAW?	Who is startled by change, but then laughs at himself, changes, and moves forward?

Johnson asks the readers to think of a change they are involved in and assess what their reaction has been. He also identifies questions we should ask as we are dealing with change:

- What are you holding on to?
- What do you need to let go of if you want to succeed in a changing situation?
- Can you change quickly enough to succeed in a rapidly changing world?
- What is keeping you from changing now? (Johnson, 1998)

To successfully initiate a change process, the nurse leader must have a vision that is consistent with the values and principles of the organization. The leader must be passionate to gain support for a shared vision and also be committed to the long haul. When implementing a change, 30% of the staff will usually support the change, 50% will be undecided, and the other 20% will resist change. Leaders often make the mistake of focusing on the resisting 20% rather than focusing on influencing the 50% who are undecided. The leader will be more successful if they can gain support from 80% of the staff rather than dwelling on the resistors to change.

Conclusion

Whether you are leading change or participating in change, you must remember that it is a process, not an event. When approaching change, leaders must be clear on the vision and make strategic choices regarding the speed of the effort, the amount of preplanning, the involvement of others, and the methods of communicating. In long-term care, strategies that address change innovation need to be implemented within a context of limited resources or culture of change. Table 5.4 outlines some ways to apply change in relation to geriatric nurse competencies in long-term care. Failure is often associated with the lack of vision, undercommunicating the vision, and failure to remove obstacles to change. A successful change takes time, communication, and involvement at all levels of the organization. It is important to remember that although change may be difficult, during times of change we may find our true direction.

5.4	Application of AACN's Geriatric Competencies in Relation to Change Theory and Process in Long-Term Care
AACN Competency:	**Goals and critical questions to ask:**
1. Critical Thinking	**Goals:** Recognize one's own and others attitudes, values and expectations about aging and their impact on care of older adults and their families; adopt the concept of individualized care as the standard of practice with older adults. **Examples of some critical questions to ask:** A. What are the health care organizations, your own, the providers and team members' attitudes and beliefs about aging? If ageist stereotypes exist are individuals and/or teams able and willing to change and adopt positive attitudes about aging and care of older adults? B. Is the health care organization and its staff responsive, flexible and reactive to the needs of the older adult and the environment? Does it place emphasis on shared values/vision?
2. Communication	**Goals:** Communicate effectively, respectfully, and compassionately with older adults and their families; recognize the biopsychosocial, functional and spiritual changes of old age. **Examples of some critical questions to ask:** A. Is the health care organization, its staff and team leaders sensitive, knowledgeable and skilled in their communication to older adults and their families? If not, are they willing and able to change in order to meet the needs of the older adult? B. Does the health care organization and its staff emphasize the importance of communication and maintaining trustworthy relationships?

(Continued)

5.4

Application of AACN's Geriatric Competencies in Relation to Change Theory and Process in Long-Term Care *(Continued)*

AACN Competency:	Goals and critical questions to ask
3. Assessment	**Goals:** Incorporate into daily practice valid and reliable tools to assess the biopsychosocial, functional and spiritual status of older adults; assess the living environment with special awareness of the biopsychosocial and functional changes common in old age; analyze the effectiveness of community resources in assisting older adults and their families to maintain independence; assess family knowledge of skills necessary to deliver care to older adult. **Examples of some critical questions to ask:** A. Do health care organizations, its team leaders and members utilize assessment tools and techniques for history taking and or physical assessment that take into consideration age-related changes, special considerations such as altered communication due to sensory impairment from associated comorbidities? If not, are they willing to adopt assessment tools that do?
4. Technical Skill	**Goals:** Adapt technical skills to meet the functional, biopsychocosial and endurance capabilities of older adults; individualize care and prevent morbidity and mortality associated with the use of physical and chemical restraints in older adults. A. Are staff able and willing to incorporate in their practice use of practical assessment tools, techniques and skills that individualize the assessment of the older adult and /or family caregiver?
5. Core Knowledge: Health Promotion, Risk Reduction, Disease Prevention	**Goals:** Prevent or reduce common risk factors that contribute to functional decline, impaired quality of life, excess disability in older adults; follow standards of care to recognize and report elder mistreatment; apply evidenced-based standards to reduce risk, screen, immunize and promote healthy lifestyles in older adults.

(Continued)

AACN Competency:	Goals and critical questions to ask
5. Core Knowledge: Health Promotion, Risk Reduction, Disease Prevention *(Continued)*	<u>Examples of some critical questions to ask</u>: A. Does the health care organization, its team leader or members utilize established national clinical guidelines for the assessment, management of various conditions unique to care of older adults and those of various cultures (example for assessment of type 2 diabetes, elder mistreatment, injury prevention, urinary incontinence and polypharmacy)? If not, are they willing and able to change the protocol by utilizing these guidelines and documents? B. Does the health care organization, its team leader or members refer to Health People 2010's guidelines for the prevention and management of diseases and conditions effecting older adults? If not, are they willing and able to change the protocol and use this document?
6. Core Knowledge: Illness and Disease Management	<u>Goals</u>: Recognize and manage geriatric syndromes common to older adults; recognize the complex interaction of acute and chronic comorbidities common to older adults. <u>Examples of some critical questions to ask</u>: A. Does the team leader empower team members to acquire the necessary state of the science knowledge in illness management and/or detection of important geriatric conditions?
7. Core Knowledge: Information and Health Care Technology	<u>Goals</u>: Use of technology to enhance older adults' function, independence and safety; facilitate communication through transitions across and between various care settings. <u>Examples of some critical questions to ask</u>: A. Does the team leader, its members utilize various technologies when working with an older clientele to improve sensory, communication or functional impairment,

(Continued)

AACN Competency:	Goals and critical questions to ask:
7. Core Knowledge: Information and Health Care Technology *(Continued)*	such as eyeglasses, use of hearing aides, canes, walkers or use of wheelchair and other adaptive devices? If not, are they able and willing to change this practice at the institution?
8. Core Knowledge: Ethics	<u>Goals:</u> Assist older adults, families and care-givers to understand and balance 'everyday' autonomy and safety decisions; apply legal and ethical principles to the complex issues that arise in care of older adults. <u>Examples of some critical questions to ask:</u> A. In the health care organization or community setting, are older adults empowered by staff to make their own decisions about health care? Are safety issues discussed openly with older adults and/or their family caregivers? B. In the health care organization or community setting, are older adults empowered by staff to maintain independence in daily living? To achieve optimal functioning? If not, are staff willing and able to make this change in the practice environment?
9. Core Knowledge: Human Diversity	<u>Goals:</u> Appreciate the influence of attitudes, roles, language, culture, race, religion, gender and lifestyle on how families and assistive personnel provide long-term care to older adults. <u>Examples of some critical questions to ask:</u> A. Does the health care facility recognize human diversity among the population served? If not, is the facility able and willing to make the necessary changes to do so?

(Continued)

5.4	**Application of AACN's Geriatric Competencies in Relation to Change Theory and Process in Long-Term Care** *(Continued)*

AACN Competency:	Goals and critical questions to ask:
10. Core Knowledge: Global Health Care	<u>Goals:</u> Evaluate differing international models of geriatric care. <u>Examples of some critical questions to ask:</u> A. Does the older adult's place of residence within long-term care recognize and or utilize health care models of geriatric care? If not, are they able and willing to take the necessary steps to do so?
11. Core Knowledge: Health Care Systems and Policy	<u>Goals:</u> Analyze the impact of an aging society on the nation's health care system; evaluate the influence of payer systems on access, availability and affordability of health care. <u>Examples of some critical questions to ask:</u> A. Are the health care services available to the older adult utilized? Are they affordable? Accessible? And are they appropriate for older adults of diverse cultures? If not, is the organization and/or its staff able and willing to take the necessary steps to make this change?
12. Core Knowledge: Provider of Care	<u>Goals:</u> Recognize the benefits of interdisciplinary teams in care of older adults; evaluate the utility of complementary and integrative health practice on health promotion and symptom management. <u>Examples of some critical questions to ask:</u> A. Does the health care organization, team leaders and health care providers recognize, utilize or explore use of complementary and integrative health care practices when caring for older adults

(Continued)

	Application of AACN's Geriatric Competencies in Relation to Change Theory and Process in Long-Term Care *(Continued)*

5.4

AACN Competency:	Goals and critical questions to ask:
12. Core Knowledge: Provider of Care *(Continued)*	of diverse cultures? If not, are they able and willing to take the steps to make this necessary change? Are structures, policy and resources available for health promotion activities such as screening and/or symptom management?
13. Core Knowledge: Designer/Manager and Coordinator of Care	<u>Goals:</u> Facilitate older adults active participation in all aspects of their own healthcare. Involve, educate and include significant others in implementing best practices for older adults; ensure quality of care commensurate with older adults vulnerability and frequency/intensity of care needs. <u>Critical questions to ask:</u> A. Are there barriers influencing the older adults participation or education about health care activities? If so, how does the health care organization and/or its team assess and manage these barriers?
14. Core Knowledge: Member of a Profession	<u>Goals:</u> Promote quality preventive and end-of-life care for older adults as essential, desirable, and integral components of nursing practice. <u>Critical questions to ask:</u> A. A. What cultural values and beliefs exist for older adults facing end-of-life care decisions? Are these values and beliefs supported within the health care organization? Within the state or territory of care? in accordance to state health policy? If not, is the health care organization able and willing to take the steps to make this change in practice/policy?

Note: Table developed by D. Gray-Miceli.
Source: American Association of Colleges of Nursing. The John A. Hartford Foundation Institute for Geriatric Nursing. (2000). *Older adults: Recommended baccalaureate competencies and curricular guidelines for geriatric nursing care.* Washington, DC: Author.

References

American Association of Colleges of Nursing. The John A. Hartford Foundation Institute for Geriatric Nursing. (2000). *Older adults: Recommended baccalaureate competencies and curricular guidelines for geriatric nursing care.* Washington, DC: Author.

Coutu, D. L. (2002, May). How resilience works. *Harvard Business Review, 80*(5), 46–55.

Havelock, R.G. (1973). The change agent's guide to innovation in education. Englewood Cliffs, NJ: Educational Technology Publications.

Johnson, S. (1998). *Who moved my cheese?* New York: G.P. Putnam's.

Karp, H.B. (1996). *The change leader.* San Francisco: Jossey-Bass Inc.

Larkin, T.J., & Larkin, S. (1996). Reaching and changing frontline employees. *Harvard Business Review, 74*, 3–12

Lewin, K. (1951). *Field theory in social science; Selected theoretical papers.* D. Cartwright, ed. New York: Harper & Row.

Lippitt, R., Watson, J., & Westley, B. (1958). *The dynamics of planned change.* New York: Harcourt, Brace and Company.

Marley, K.M., & Reck, D.L. (2006). The role of nursing leadership in clinical transformation. *Nurse Leader, 4*(6), 29–33.

McDaniel, R. R. (1996). Strategic leadership: A view from quantum and chaos theories. In W.J. Duncan, P. Ginter, & L. Swayne, (eds.), *Handbook of health care management* (p. 8). Oxford, England: Basil Blackwell Publishing.

Rogers, E. M. (1995). *Diffusion of innovations* (4th ed.). New York: Simon and Schuster.

Senge, P. M. (1990). *The fifth discipline: The art and practice of the learning organization.* New York: Doubleday Currency.

Tiffany, C. R., & Lutjens, L. R. J. (1998). *Planned change theories for nursing: Review, analysis, and implications.* Thousand Oaks, CA: Sage Publications.

Yoder-Wise, P. S. (1999). *Leading and managing in nursing* (2nd ed.). St. Louis, MO: Mosby.

Your ID _____   RN _____ Non RN _____
Today's Date ____/____/____   Facility: _____

Change Theory and Process

Post-test (circle one)

Please circle T if the statement is True and F is the statement is False.

1. Everyone's initial response to change is anger.

   T   F

2. Two requirements for effective individual change are willingness and anxiety related to potential job loss.

   T   F

3. It is important for a leader to spend energy and time on all employees, especially those most resistant to change.

   T   F

4. Individual responses to change can progress from denial to resistance to exploration and then commitment.

   T   F

5. When individuals are in a resistant mode, it is important for the leader to continue to give them information and direction.

   T   F

6. During times of change, resilience is perceived as a negative attribute.

   T   F

7. To lead change a leader must be passionate, have a vision, and accept stumbles, falls, and move forward.

   T   F

Please circle the item that is not a characteristic.

8. Characteristics of change include all of the following EXCEPT:
   a. Evokes multiple responses
   b. It's inevitable and ever-present
   c. Slow paced and requires consensus
   d. Can be disruptive, intrusive, and upsets status quo

Participant Evaluation Form

Change Theory and Process

Today's Date ___/___/___   Facility: _____

Please circle the best response.

Example: Strongly Disagree   Disagree   Agree   Strongly Agree
             1   2   3   4

At the end of the presentation I can:

1. Discuss the importance of the change process in health care services.

Strongly Disagree   Disagree   Agree   Strongly Agree
         1   2   3   4

2. Discuss the positive and negative human responses to change.

Strongly Disagree   Disagree   Agree   Strongly Agree
         1   2   3   4

3. Be more aware of the impact of change and your personal response to change.

Strongly Disagree   Disagree   Agree   Strongly Agree
         1   2   3   4

4. Understand the role of the leader in facilitating change.

Strongly Disagree   Disagree   Agree   Strongly Agree
         1   2   3   4

5. Discuss the concepts of leadership and change.

Strongly Disagree   Disagree   Agree   Strongly Agree
         1   2   3   4

6. Identify some of the barriers to implementing effective change.

Strongly Disagree	Disagree	Agree	Strongly Agree
1	2	3	4

7. Understand the concept of resilience and its importance during change.

Strongly Disagree	Disagree	Agree	Strongly Agree
1	2	3	4

8. This program will help me work better with other staff.

Strongly Disagree	Disagree	Agree	Strongly Agree
1	2	3	4

Overall, I rate:

9. This program

Poor	Fair	Good	Excellent
1	2	3	4

10. The case scenario

Poor	Fair	Good	Excellent	not applicable
1	2	3	4	n/a

11. Speaker _____ [insert name]

Poor	Fair	Good	Excellent
1	2	3	4

12. This program would be better if:

13. What other leadership topics would be helpful to you in the future?

Principles of Education

Developing Cultural Competence in Long-Term Care Nursing
Pre-test (circle one)

Please circle the *best* answer among the items listed below.

1. Culturally competent care is best defined as:

   a. The use of one's personal experience to treat patients and staff.
   b. Using the institution's cultural staff to meet the needs of the patients and other staff.
   c. Understanding another culture that is different from one's own culture and using that knowledge to treat everyone else the same way.
   d. A set of skills, knowledge, and attitudes that respect the values of others when rendering care, even when it conflicts with one's own personal beliefs or values.

2. Health care organizations need to provide culturally competent care because:

   a. It is documented in the Constitution of the United States.
   b. Many people cannot speak English or have limited proficiency in English.
   c. Of changing demographics, reports of health disparities, current legislative protocols, and evidence of positive patient outcomes.
   d. Organizations will be able to receive more money from the government.

3. Cultural sensitivity is best described as:

   a. Being sensitive and respectful of the values and beliefs of others, which may or may not conflict with one's own values and beliefs.
   b. Knowing that cultural differences and similarities exist within and between groups without assigning value to the differences.

c. A process of changing one's personal values to those of others.

d. Trying to learn another language so one can help the patients.

4. What is the first step to becoming a culturally competent health care provider?

a. Talking with someone from another culture all the time.
b. Self-appraisal of one's own cultural values and beliefs.
c. Listening and learning languages other than English.
d. Taking classes to learn all the possible cultures in the world.

5. Choose the five strategies for bridging the cultural health gap, as outlined by Berlin and Fowkes.

a. Assess, Explain, Evaluate, Implement, and Observe (AEEIO)
b. Explain, Negotiate, Decide, Overcome, and Sign (ENDOS)
c. Listen, Explain, Acknowledge, Recommend, and Negotiate (LEARN)
d. Assess, Decide, Implement, Evaluate, and Report (ADIER)

6. Which one of the following would not be an effective strategy for cross-cultural communication?

a. Having respect for the values of others
b. Seeing differences in others as primarily weaknesses
c. Seeing differences as strengths rather than weaknesses
d. Recognizing unfamiliar situations as interesting instead of annoying

7. Communication about health beliefs and practices of residents/patients requires that culturally competent providers:

a. Discuss the meaning of health and illness, its etiology, and cultural-specific concerns.
b. Provide opportunity for patients to describe their symptoms and approaches for coping with stressors.
c. Discuss the role of the family during sickness.
d. All of the above

Match the following terms on the *left* to the correct definitions on the *right*.

Term		Definition
8. **Ethnicity**	_____	A. Belief that race is the primary determinant of human traits and capabilities and the inherent superiority of a particular race.
9. **Stereotype**	_____	B. Intentional or unintentional actions against a group or individuals based on gender, racial groups, ethnicity, sexual orientation, or education.
10. **Racism**	_____	C. Self-defined affiliation with a specific group or subgroup that shares common cultural heritage due to history, customs, and language passed on from generation to generation.
11. **Discrimination**	_____	D. A fixed picture or set mental image that is used to represent all people from a group.
12. **Cultural Knowledge**	_____	E. Familiarization with cultural history, values, and belief systems of the members of another group.

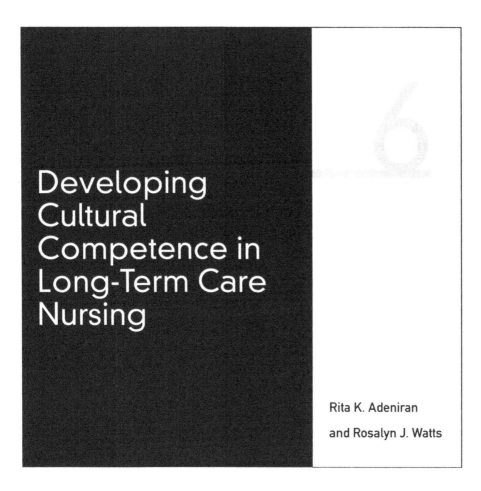

Developing Cultural Competence in Long-Term Care Nursing

Rita K. Adeniran
and Rosalyn J. Watts

Changing demographics in a pluralistic society of multiethnic racial groups is a daunting challenge for providers throughout the spectrum of health care delivery systems. In long-term care settings, registered nurses in leadership positions are challenged to advance the agenda for the delivery of culturally competent health care. The comprehensive report of the Institute of Medicine (2003) clearly documented that unequal treatment in health care persists for racial and ethnic minorities. The U.S. Department of Health and Human Services (2001) has outlined the national standards for the delivery of the Culturally and Linguistically Appropriate Services (CLAS). The notion of the word *competence* implies the ability to function effectively. Thus, cultural competence does not occur in isolation or just within the context of the provider–patient clinical encounter. It involves the vision of the leadership group, organizational commitment, and definitive strategies to eliminate systemic barriers in health care delivery for multicultural vulnerable patients. When professional nurses and support staff, such as LPNs and certified nursing assistants (CNAs) or direct care workers, begin the process of developing greater sensitivity, knowledge, and skill about the dimensions of cultural diversity in their patient populations, it is anticipated that these providers are more likely to respond in an appropriate manner during the clinical scenario thereby bridging the provider–patient cultural gap.

> . . . cultural competence does not occur in isolation or just within the context of the provider–patient clinical encounter. It involves the vision of the leadership group, organizational commitment, and definitive strategies to eliminate systemic barriers in health care delivery for multicultural vulnerable patients.

Purpose

The purpose of this chapter is to provide a framework for cultural competence education for professional nurses who work in long-term care facilities. It is anticipated that these individuals in leadership positions will develop the requisite cultural sensitivity, knowledge, and skills to disseminate this information to other RNs, LPNs, CNAs, and those providing care in extended care settings. By the end of this module these nurses should be better able to:

- Describe the characteristics of cultural competence in nursing,
- Outline evidence of the need for delivery of culturally competent care health,
- Identify strategies for facilitating cross-cultural communication with patients and families,
- Identify tools to support the delivery of culturally competent health care services, and
- Apply the principles of cultural competence with analyses of case scenarios in long-term care.

What Is Cultural Competence in Nursing?

The expert panel of the American Academy of Nursing defines cultural competence as "having the knowledge, understanding and skills about a diverse cultural group that allows the health care provider to provide culturally acceptable care" (Giger et al., 2007, p. 100). Theorists and clinicians describing this phenomenon fully recognize that cultural competence is a multidimensional construct consisting of cultural awareness, knowledge, and skill acquisition (Campinha-Bacote, 2002; Giger & Davidhizar, 2004; Leininger, 2002; Purnell, 2002; Spector, 2004). For the providers, cultural competence is not an end point or single event but a developmental process of becoming (Campinha-Bacote, 2002). There are various definitions for cultural competence in the relevant literature, even though none has been accepted as the "gold standard" definition. Some common themes evident in most definitions include:

- Assessing and understanding one's own cultural values and beliefs. In other words, *provider's self-reflection.*
- Acknowledging and respecting the patient's culture, value systems, beliefs, and behavioral standards. In other words, *respect* for the patients different cultures.
- Recognizing that cultural difference is not synonymous with cultural inferiority but rather identifying with cultural difference as a relationship between two cultural perspectives. In other words, *awareness* of the existence of diverse cultures and value systems.
- A willingness to learn about other cultures including the patient's culture. In other words, practice of *humility and the craving for knowledge about different cultures.*
- Adapting optimal health care delivery services to an acceptable cultural framework. In other words, utilizing *skill* to successfully navigate through the different patient cultures resulting in optimal outcomes.

In the simplest terms, cultural competence can be defined as the ability of the nurse or health care provider to deliver health care services using a framework that is congruent with the patient's cultural health beliefs. During the clinical encounter, cultural competence can be achieved by the provider's ability to create an environment where the patient will be comfortable in sharing important information about cultural health beliefs. In the long run, the provider will be able to present appropriate care planning and interventions, ultimately improving adherence to treatment and health outcomes. It is left for the provider to understand the unique needs of the patient and provide care congruent with the patient health

During the clinical encounter, cultural competence can be achieved by the provider's ability to create an environment where the patient will be comfortable in sharing important information about cultural health beliefs.

beliefs. Research and expert reports indicate that patients are more likely to adhere to a provider's plan of care when the care is congruent with the patient's cultural health beliefs and patient input is included when designing the plan of care (Betancourt, Green, & Carrillo, 2002; Campinha-Bacote, Betancourt, Carrillo, & Green, 1999; Di Clemente & Wingwood, 1995; Ngo-Metzger, Telfair, & Sorkin, 2006).

It would be naïve to assume that culturally competent care can be achieved once a provider is willing and has acquired the knowledge and skill necessary to deliver culturally competent care. Variables that affect patient outcomes expand beyond just the provider's willingness, knowledge, and skill. Organizational structures, leadership, and the environment where the provider practices all have a major role in ensuring that patients receive culturally competent care. Organizations that recognize, embrace, and value the importance of culturally competent health care services set the stage for their clinicians to deliver care that is culturally appropriate. Structures, policies, procedure arrangements, and resources to support the practice of culturally competent care must be in place to sustain appropriate clinician practice. Therefore, it is no wonder that one of the most widely used and applicable definitions of cultural competence includes the role of the health care organization. The HHS Office of Minority Health (OMH) Web site defines cultural competency as:

> Cultural and linguistic competence is a set of congruent behaviors, attitudes, and policies that come together in a system, agency, or among professionals that enables effective work in cross-cultural situations. "Culture" refers to integrated patterns of human behavior that include the language, thoughts, communications, actions, customs, beliefs, values, and institutions of racial, ethnic, religious, or social groups. "Competence" implies having the capacity to function effectively as an individual and an organization within the context of the cultural beliefs, behaviors, and needs presented by consumers and their communities. (U.S. Department of Health and Human Services, n.d.)

This definition has been adopted by the HHS and OMH in launching the Cultural and Linguistic Appropriate Services (CLAS) standards in March 2001 (U.S. Department of Health and Human

Services, 2001). Adoption of a culturally competent approach further allows professional nurses to deliver all of the essential core competencies for providing high-quality care to older adults and their families outlined by the American Association of Colleges of Nursing (AACN).

Need for Delivery of Culturally Competent Care

Changing Demographics in America

As the U.S. demographics continues to change, with ethnic minority populations growing at rates surpassing the rest of the population, cultural competence has become an essential tool for all clinicians, specifically nurses, who are the single largest providers of health care services. As such, professional nurses provide continuous care to older adult patients 24 hours daily. In this practice setting, it is fitting and appropriate that culturally competent care be delivered by professional nurses to their patients. According to the U.S. Census Bureau, by 2050, the U.S. population distribution will be as follows: White, 52.5%; Hispanic, 22.5%; African American, 14.4%; Asian/Pacific Islander, 9.7%; and Native American, 0.9% (U.S. Census Bureau, 2000). This data shows that current minority groups increase in size and will become the majority in the near future. Of note, strong evidence exists about the long-standing disparities that exist against racial and ethnic minorities.

Evidence of Disparities in Health Care

The Institute of Medicine (IOM) reports *Unequal Treatment: Confronting Racial and Ethnic Disparities in Health Care* (2003), which also appears in *Crossing the Quality Chasm: A New Health System for the 21st Century* (Institute of Medicine, 2001), illustrates the issue of lower quality of care experienced mainly by minority patients across a wide range of conditions, even after adjusting for health insurance coverage and socioeconomic status. In this report, the definition of disparity, either health status disparity or health care disparity, is further explicated.

Health status disparities occur when different racial groups suffer disproportionately from a number of health issues because of genetic and society reasons. For instance, African Americans are more prone to suffer disproportionately from obesity than their

Health care disparities, on the other hand, are defined as "racial or ethnic differences in the quality of health care that are not due to access-related factors or clinical needs, preferences, and appropriateness of intervention."

White counterparts, and Caucasians are more likely to suffer illnesses such as cystic fibrosis. Health care disparities, on the other hand, are defined as "racial or ethnic differences in the quality of health care that are not due to access-related factors or clinical needs, preferences, and appropriateness of intervention" (Institute of Medicine, 2003, pp. 3–4). Health care disparities, in a simple language, mean some people get better treatment than others just because of their racial or ethnic background.

An unimaginable crisis awaits the health care delivery system if appropriate attention is not directed to eliminating the current health care disparities. According to the U.S. Department of Commerce, Minority Business Development Agency (1999), the U.S. population is projected to increase from 263 million in 1995 to 394 million by 2050. With racially and ethnically diverse populations accounting for 90% of the growth, one can only imagine the economic and human loss to society if health care disparities continue in the health care system.

Burden of Disparities in Health Care

Health care disparities are burdensome and costly to both individuals and society in general. Even though the economic implications of disparities are yet to be quantified, the cost of providing health care will be greatly influenced by the effectiveness of care that growing minority populations receive.

Factors contributing to health disparities are complex: comprising societal factors, environmental factors, and structural factors, including the lack of knowledge and skill on the part of the clinician in providing culturally appropriate care. In their research, Betancourt, Green, and Carrillo (2002) reported three levels of social cultural barriers that significantly contribute to racial and ethnic disparities. The following paragraphs discuss in detail each type of barrier that exists at the various levels: organizational, structural, and clinical.

Organizational Barriers. The availability and acceptability of health care services for racial and ethnic minorities correlates with the degree to which health care leadership and workforce reflect the racial composition of the general population. In other words, the health care workforce should reflect a microcosm of the general population. Currently, the U.S. health care workforce does not mirror the patient population served. As an example, according to the U.S. Census Bureau (2005), minorities represent 33% of the U.S. population, yet African Americans comprise only 4.2% of the RN population, Hispanic/Latinos only 1.7%, and Asians only 3.1% (U.S. Department of Health and Human Services, 2004). This evidence illustrates one of the organizational barriers contributing to health care disparities in the workplace.

Structural Barriers. Vulnerable populations, such as the ethnic populations, and economically disadvantaged populations suffer in an environment where economic forces alone may dominate health care delivery. Examples of such are lack of health care insurance for any reason, or lack of interpreters for limited English proficiency patients. Additionally, navigating the bureaucratic intake and referral process for patients with limited English is a challenge that also contributes to health care disparities.

Clinical Barriers. Effective communication between the provider and patient is critical for the delivery of safe effective health care services. A clinical barrier occurs when sociocultural differences exist between the provider and the patient. If these differences are not fully explored or understood, or when there is a communication gap due to language difference, ineffective communication occurs. Further, clinical practices solely based on the provider's illness explanatory model, in addition to unconscious stereotypes or bias, can lead to less than optimal health outcomes (Cooper & Powe, 2004; Institute of Medicine, 2003, 2004; Kleinman, Eisenberg, & Good, 1978; Leah, Jacobs, Chen, & Sunita, 2007; Wynia & Matiasek, 2006).

Solutions to Minimize the Effects of Barriers That Exist in Health Care

Culturally competent health care services have been identified as one of the major strategies to eliminate health care disparities. This is a promising solution whose origin is reflected in various nursing position statements and recommendations by the AACN for core competencies in geriatric health care. According to Anderson and colleagues, "When clients do not understand what their healthcare providers are telling them, and providers either do not speak the client's language or are insensitive to cultural differences, the quality of health care can be compromised" (2003, p. 1).

The American Nurses Association (ANA) position statement on cultural diversity in nursing practice underscores the importance of cultural competence in health care delivery with this position statement:

> Knowledge of cultural diversity is vital at all levels of nursing practice. Ethnocentric approaches to nursing practice are ineffective in meeting health and nursing needs of diverse cultural groups of clients. Knowledge about cultures and their impact on interactions with health care is essential for nurses, whether they are practicing in a clinical setting, education, research or administration. Cultural diversity addresses racial and ethnic differences, however, these concepts or features of the human experience are not synonymous. The changing demographics of the nation as reflected in the 1990 census will increase the cultural diversity of the U.S. population by the year 2000, and what have therefore been called minority groups will, on the whole constitute a national majority. (ANA, 1991)

According to Anderson and colleagues, "When clients do not understand what their healthcare providers are telling them, and providers either do not speak the client's language or are insensitive to cultural differences, the quality of health care can be compromised" (2003, p. 1).

Imperatives for Better Health Outcomes: Excellence and Cost of Care

Cultural competence is an essential ingredient in quality health care. Providers' cultural competence has been closely linked to better health outcomes, higher quality of health care services, increased access to health care services, and more satisfied health care consumers. In their analysis of evidence-based research studies, Goode, Dunne, and Bronheim (2006) reported three studies that used comparison or control groups utilizing patient education approaches designed with and for the intended audience and consistent with the audience's values, beliefs, and preferred ways of getting information. These studies demonstrated significantly increased behavior changes compared with either no intervention or interventions that were not culturally competent (Goode, Dunne, & Bronheim, 2006). Additionally, in the same report, three other studies that had pre- and post-intervention data on the effects of culturally competent interventions reported significantly improved outcomes in terms of physiologic measures associated with better long-term outcomes in diabetes.

The culturally competent clinician is also more satisfied with their job and able to work more efficiently and effectively in cross-cultural situations. Health care organizations have never been challenged to increase their market share until fairly recently. In an era of capitation, technology, enhanced consumerism, and outcome-based payor systems, health care organizations are now challenged to attract and gain loyalty of patients as well as health care professionals. Older adult consumers "shop" for health care services just as they do for other services. As recipients of health care, older adult patients are more likely to return for care or refer other peers to the health care organization where they received satisfactory health care services. Health care organizations can also leverage their market share (patient volume), clinicians' level of expertise, and the "organizational cultural competence" in negotiating payments by third-party insurance providers. There is evidence that culturally competent clinicians are less likely to be litigated, a fact that appeals to third-party insurance providers and organizations. Some studies indicate that the patients of physicians who are frequently sued had the most complaints about communication (Levinson, Roter, Mullooly, Dull, & Frankel, 1997; Virshup, Oppenberg, & Coleman, 1999). Furthermore, mandates exist for health care organizations and health care providers to communicate with limited English proficiency patients and non-English speaking patients in the patient primary language CLAS (U.S. Department of Health and Human Services, 2001). The Language Assess Services (LAS), the second theme of the three themes of the CLAS standards, mandates organizations and providers to communicate with patients in their primary language. Those providers and organizations who fail to comply with these mandates are at greater risk for litigation in addition to losing federal funding. These are strong incentives for change in current practice patterns.

As recipients of health care, older adult patients are more likely to return for care or refer other peers to the health care organization where they received satisfactory health care services.

Legislative, Regulatory, and Accrediting Imperatives

Different regulatory legislatives and creditor imperatives serve as incentives to encourage and empower health care organizations and providers to provide cultural competence services to their increasingly diverse patient population. The bullet points highlight some of these imperatives:

- Title VI of the Civil Rights Act of 1964 legislation mandates "no person in the United States shall, on ground of race, color, or national origin, be excluded from participation in, be denied the benefits of, or be subjected to discrimination under any program or activity receiving federal financial assistance."
- The Joint Commission of Accreditation of Healthcare Organizations (JCAHO) necessitates health care organizations to demonstrate practices that incorporate the patients' culture into their plan of care.
- The American Nurses Credentialing Center (ANCC) requires that health care organizations recognize and respect the cultural values of their patients and workforce in order to obtain magnet status.

Above and beyond the economic and legal rationales, culturally competent health care service is the right thing to do from an ethical perspective. Patients interface with clinicians at a time of potential vulnerability and clinicians must focus on the ways that patients can be in the best position to respond to care and treatment. Culturally competent care creates the context in which vulnerabilites due to language or cultural differences can be minimized for the benefit of the patient (Meleis, 2005).

Provider Strategies for Providing Culturally Competent Care

Conceptual Models as Framework for Cultural Competence Practice

Different theories, models, and frameworks exist to guide clinicians and organizations to facilitate the practice of and delivery of culturally competent health care services. Although we will primarily discuss Campinha-Bacote's Process of Cultural Competence in this chapter, Table 6.1 briefly discusses some of the other models and framework guiding clinicians in delivering culturally appropriate care. Campinha-Bacote's model (2002) titled *The Process of Cultural Competence in the Delivery of Healthcare Services* provides an excellent framework for clinical practice. It views cultural competence as an ongoing process in which the health care professionals continuously strive to achieve the ability to work effectively within the cultural context of the client, individual, family, and community. This model requires health care professionals to see themselves as *becoming* culturally competent rather than *being* culturally competent.

6.1 Examples of Cultural Competence Models	
Model	**Brief Description of the Model**
Purnell, L. (2002)	Larry Purnell presents his model of cultural competence as an organizing framework for guiding cultural competence development among multidisciplinary health care professionals. He reported that a culturally competent health care provider develops awareness of their existence, sensations, and environment without letting these factors have an undue effect on the care that is provided (Purnell, 2002). The model challenges health care professionals to continuously "raise awareness" through consciousness. Increasing one's consciousness of cultural diversity improves the possibilities for providers to provide culturally competent care. The model identified four stages in the continuum of cultural competence, and that the provider's level of awareness or consciousness regarding interactions with diverse cultural groups determines what stage that provider can function at as well as the level of competence. The four stages are not concretely linear because providers may be at any of the stages in any clinical encounter. He claims that providers are always in the process for "becoming" culturally competent because the process is not necessarily linear nor an endpoint. Providers progress from unconscious incompetence to unconscious competence. Following are the four Purnell stages of cultural competence:

(Continued)

Model	Brief Description of the Model
	Unconsciously Incompetent: This is the stage where the provider lacks knowledge and awareness of the differences that exist in value and cultures between themselves and the patient due to ethnocentric beliefs. Ethnocentric beliefs force providers to use their knowledge and culture as the standard for treating their patients. The provider may be thinking that they are doing the right thing to help the patient, because they are providing the best possible care. Even though the clinician is making the best biomedical decision possible for the patient's situation, the intervention or choice of treatment may disgust the patient because it is out of line with the patient's cultural health beliefs, which may lead to no adherence. Culture is largely unconscious and has powerful influences on health and illness. Health care providers must recognize, respect, and integrate clients' cultural beliefs and practices into health care planning and interventions. Thus, the provider must be culturally aware, culturally sensitive, and have some degree of cultural competence to be effective.
	Consciously Incompetent: Conscious incompetence is being aware that one is lacking knowledge about another culture; the provider understands and knows that the patient culture plays a major role in whether the patient follows through with planned intervention. At this level, the providers just do not know how to assess the patient's cultural values or plan appropriate culturally competent interventions.
	Consciously Competent: Conscious competence occurs when the provider has acquired some knowledge and skills about caring for patients from different cultures. The provider uses generalization as the beginning point of assessment, verifying the patient's unique culture, and providing culturally specific intervention. This is the point where the clinician is cautious and does the best to provide care that is congruent with the patient's cultural values. The provider sometimes may feel

(Continued)

Model	Brief Description of the Model
	the need to say the right thing. Please note that politically correct statements without honest commitments to the principles of cultural competence are NOT synonymous with competence.
	Unconsciously Competent: Unconscious competence occurs when the provider is able to automatically provide culturally competent care to clients of diverse cultures. Unconscious competence is difficult to accomplish and potentially dangerous because individual differences exist within specific cultural groups, and there are more variations within a group than across groups. Providers cannot assume that because they come from the same ethnic background as a client, that they and the patient share similar cultural values.
Leininger, M. (2002)	Leininger's Sunrise Model suggests the worldview and social structure of the client are important areas to explore using the following seven dimensions:
	(1) Cultural values and life-ways; (2) Religious, philosophical, and spiritual beliefs; (3) Economic factors; (4) Educational factors; (5) Technological factors; (6) Kinship and social ties; and (7) Political and legal factors. Leininger informed that the Western medical model fails to explore cultural patterns of illness, and request health care professionals to develop the skills, knowledge, and patience to explore and validate what the patient cultural health care values and beliefs. Information obtained about each of the dimensions can guide plan of treatment and interventions. The Sunrise Model advised providers to base their intervention on information gathered from the assessment. Suggesting that this guidance can occur in a variety of ways: cultural care preservation and/or maintenance, cultural care accommodation and/or negotiation, and cultural care repatterning and/or restructuring. She declares that the Sunrise Model for assessing patients can provide comprehensive information for providing culturally sensitive care.

(Continued)

6.1	Examples of Cultural Competence Models *(Continued)*
Model	**Brief Description of the Model**
Giger & Davidhizar (2004)	Giger and Davidhizar present a transcultural assessment model to assist health care professionals in assessing patients from diverse cultures that focuses on six factors: (1) Communication, (2) Space, (3) Time, (4) Social organization, (5) Environmental control, and (6) Biological variations. Giger and Davidhizar asserts that health care professionals should receive training on how to use these factors to assess the health beliefs and practices because health care values and beliefs may impact on how an individual responds to follow-through with treatment plans and education. Appropriate use of the model is believed to have the capability of helping health care professionals provide culturally competent care.
Cross, Bazron, Dennis, & Isaccs (1989)	Cross, et al. offer a theoretical approach in which cultural competence is seen as a process or continuum whereby an individual's view of other cultures is along a six-level continuum, from destructive to proficient. Cross, et al. also identified conditions that must be in place for individuals to progress along the six possible points on this continuum: (1) Cultural destructiveness, (2) Cultural incapacity, (3) Cultural blindness, (4) Cultural pre-competence, (5) Cultural competence, and (6) Cultural proficiency. The conditions that must exist in order for professionals to move along this continuum are: Valuing diversity, understanding one's own culture, consciousness of the dynamics that occur when cultures interact, internalizing cultural knowledge, and developing adaptations to diversity. According to Cross, et al., each of the conditions must function at every level of the health care system in order for that system to provide culturally competent care.

Assumptions of Campinha-Bacote Model of Cultural Competence

Dr. Campinha-Bacote identified the following as fundamentals that can serve to guide clinicians in the delivery of culturally competent care:

- Cultural competence is a process, not an event; a journey, not a destination; dynamic, not static; and involves the paradox of knowing.
- Cultural competence is an essential component in providing effective and culturally responsive nursing care to all clients.
- All encounters are cultural encounters.
- There is more variation within cultural groups than across cultural groups.
- There is a direct relationship between health care professionals' level of cultural competence and their ability to provide culturally responsive health care services.
- The process of cultural competence consists of five interrelated constructs: cultural desire, cultural awareness, cultural knowledge, cultural skill, and cultural encounters. The key pivotal construct is cultural desire.

The following paragraphs further discuss each of these constructs in detail:

Cultural Desire: Cultural desire is defined as the motivation of the health care provider to "want to, rather than have to, engage in the process of becoming culturally aware, culturally knowledgeable, culturally skillful, and familiar with cultural encounters" (Campinha-Bacote, 2002, p. 182). The motivation is genuine and authentic with no hidden agendas because the goal is not to offer comments that are politically correct; rather it reflects the provider's inner experiences, thoughts, and willingness to care in a culturally competent manner.

Cultural Awareness: Cultural awareness is the self-examination and in-depth exploration of one's own cultural background (Campinha-Bacote, 2002, p. 182). It is the conscious cognitive and emotional process of getting to know yourself: your personality, your values, your beliefs, your professional knowledge standards, your ethics, and the

The ability to understand one's self sets the stage for integrating new knowledge related to cultural differences into the professional's knowledge base and perceptions of health interventions. Even then, traces of ethnocentrism may unconsciously pervade one's attitudes and behavior.

impact of these factors on the various roles played when interacting with individuals who are different from yourself. The ability to understand one's self sets the stage for integrating new knowledge related to cultural differences into the professional's knowledge base and perceptions of health interventions. Even then, traces of ethnocentrism may unconsciously pervade one's attitudes and behavior.

Cultural Knowledge: Cultural knowledge "is the process of seeking and obtaining a sound educational foundation about diverse cultural and ethnic groups" (Campinha-Bacote, 2002, p. 182). Lavizzo-Mourey and Mackenzie (1996) suggest that health care professionals must focus on the integration of three specific issues in obtaining cultural knowledge: (1) health-related beliefs, practices and cultural values; (2) disease incidence and prevalence; and (3) treatment efficacy. It is unrealistic to expect health care providers to have in-depth knowledge of all cultures, but it is realistic to expect a broad perspective. It is possible to have a broad understanding of the patient's unique cultural beliefs and values and adjust your behavior accordingly. Acquiring cultural knowledge encompasses the understanding that behaviors and responses may be viewed by different cultures in many ways. Examples of such are: interpretation of illness, death rituals, role of family in care, effectiveness and values of different types of interventions, and religious beliefs. Additionally, providers can enhance their skill in providing culturally competent care through their understanding of cultural bound illnesses or syndromes to help maintain diagnostic clarity. Leff (1981) defines *cultural bound syndrome* as features of an illness that vary from culture to culture. For example, Suto (fright) and Mal ojo (evil eye) are cultural bound syndromes noted in the Hispanic/Latino population of how specific cultural groups respond to certain medication due to genetic mappings.

Additionally, providers can enhance their skill in providing culturally competent care through their understanding of cultural bound illnesses or syndromes to help maintain diagnostic clarity. Leff (1981) defines *cultural bound syndrome* as features of an illness that vary from culture to culture.

Cultural Skill: According to Campinha-Bacote (2002, p. 182), cultural skill "is the ability to collect relevant cultural data regarding the clients' presenting problem as well as accurately perform a culturally based physical assessment." Dr. Campinha-Bacote (2002) discussed an integrated model of conducting cultural assessments. She asked clinicians to:

- Review several cultural assessment tools.
- Consider the provider's discipline or practice area in conducting the assessment.
- Consider personal assets and liabilities as an interviewer.
- Incorporate selected questions from specific cultural assessment tools to augment the provider's skills in obtaining cultural relevant data.

Some of the assessment tools that can be used to enhance clinicians' skills in collecting cultural relevant data are further discussed in the "Clinical Guidelines for Obtaining a Cultural Specific History" section of this chapter.

Cultural Encounter: Cultural encounter "is the process that encourages the health care provider to directly engage in cross-cultural interactions with clients from culturally diverse backgrounds" (Campinha-Bacote, 2002, p. 182). Dr. Campinha asserts that every encounter is cross cultural, and she encourages health care professionals to interact with patients from diverse cultures because these experiences will expose them to diverse cultural belief systems and increase their understanding and confidence in planning care intervention.

Campinha-Bacote (2002, p. 181) model assumptions are:

1. Cultural competence is a process, not an event.
2. Cultural competence consists of five constructs: cultural awareness, cultural knowledge, cultural skill, cultural encounters, and cultural desire.
3. There is more variation within ethnic groups than across ethnic groups (intra-ethnic variation).
4. There is a direct relationship between the level of competence of health care providers and their ability to provide culturally responsive health care services.
5. Cultural competence is an essential component in rendering effective and culturally responsive services to culturally and ethnically diverse clients.

In her model, Dr. Campinha-Bacote (2002) emphasizes the importance of seeing cultural competence as a journey in which the clinician is always in the process of becoming culturally competent and never reaching a destination. This is because of the very dynamic nature of culture as well as the many variables that exist about cultures. No two individuals will exhibit the same culture at all times.

Clinical Guidelines for Obtaining a Cultural Specific History

Berlin and Fowkes (1983) utilize the mnemonic LEARN as a guide to clinicians in appropriately assessing patients to deliver culturally competent health care services. They suggest using a mnemonic can help the clinician understand the patent illness model of explanation as well as support them in designing appropriate intervention. Table 6.2 highlights each letter of the mnemonic and what it means in the processes.

The RESPECT mnemonic was developed by the Boston University Residence Program in Internal Medicine, Diversity Curriculum Task Force, but it was published by Bigby (2003), who describes how clinicians can reach out to provide culturally competent care to their patients. Details of this mnemonic are explained in Table 6.3.

Tools to Support Culturally Competent Health Care Services

Health care professionals can equip themselves with the following recommendations as tools to help them provide culturally competent services to diverse consumers of health care services.

Clinicians should strive to understand how residents, especially older adults:

- Define life processes;
- Define health, illness, and its etiology;
- Maintain wellness;
- Define pain, get motivated, and cope;
- Make health care decisions; and
- Define respect.

Clinicians should also strive to:

- Acquire knowledge about and understand other cultures,
- See unfamiliar situations as interesting instead of annoying,

6.2 The LEARN Mnemonic

The LEARN Mnemonic	Description of Use
"L"	The "L" portion of the mnemonic stands for "Listen," with sympathy and understand the patient's perception of the problem. It emphasizes the need for clinicians to listen to the patient's concept of the causes, prognosis' expected outcomes, as well as the healing modalities that the patient considers appropriate.
"E"	The "E" portion of the mnemonic stands for "Explain." At this point, the clinician explains their perception of the problem. This section stresses the importance of clinician just communicating the biomedical understanding of the cause, not necessarily imposing their understanding. The patient should be given the opportunity to understand the biomedical explanation
"A"	The "A" portion of the mnemonic stands for "Acknowledge." Clinicians should acknowledge and discuss the differences and similarities of both models of illness explanation. The clinician at this point acknowledges the patient explanation of the illness while discussing treatment. Additionally, the patient and clinician have the opportunity to learn the potential conflict that may arise due to the planned treatments and have opportunity to discuss and sort out things.
"R"	The "R" portion of the mnemonic stands for "Recommend Treatment." The providers' understanding of the patient cultural health beliefs allows the provider to be able to recommend treatments that the patient is most likely to adhere to.
"N"	The "N" portion of the mnemonic stands for "Negotiate Agreement." The patient may not always agree to the clinicians' recommendations, but the clinician can negotiate agreement within the boundaries of the bio-medical model in order to incorporate the patient cultural need.

6.3 The RESPECT Mnemonic

The RESPECT Mnemonic	Description
R. Rapport	▪ Connect on a social level ▪ See the patient point of view ▪ Consciously attempt to suspend judgment ▪ Recognize and avoid making assumptions
E. Empathy	▪ Remember that the patient has come to you for help ▪ Seek out and understand the patient's rationale for his/her behaviors or illness ▪ Verbally acknowledge and legitimize the patient's feelings
S. Support	▪ Ask about and try to understand barriers to care and compliance ▪ Help the patient overcome barriers ▪ Involve family members if appropriate ▪ Reassure the patient that you are and will be available to help
P. Partnership	▪ Be flexible with regard to issues of control ▪ Negotiate roles when necessary ▪ Stress that you will be working together to address medical problems
E. Explanations	▪ Check often for understanding ▪ Use verbal clarification techniques
C. Cultural Competence	▪ Respect the patient and his/her culture and beliefs ▪ Understand that the patient's view of you may be defined by ethnic and cultural stereotype ▪ Be aware of your own biases and preconceptions ▪ Know your limitations in addressing medical issues across cultures ▪ Recognize your personal styles and recognize when it may not be working with a given patient
T. Trust	▪ Self disclosure may be an issue for some patients who are not accustomed to Western medical approaches ▪ Take the necessary time and consciously work to establish trust

■ Practice flexible thinking and active listening, and
■ See differences as strengths rather than weaknesses.

Clinicians should strive to also identify and become aware of some generic barriers to providing culturally competent care, including:

■ Ethnocentrism: the belief that one's own cultural values and beliefs are superior and better than others;
■ Prejudice: prejudging the patient.
■ Stereotyping: a fixed mental picture about certain cultural groups, often negative, not considering individual differences;
■ Discrimination: biased against an individual or group on the basis of their cultural group such as race, ethnicity, class, sexual orientation, age, or disabilities;
■ Racism: actions and decisions based on the superiority of a specific cultural group over another. Often the privileged group excising superiority over the disadvantage group; and
■ Ignorance: making decisions, hypothesizing due to lack of knowledge.

Conclusion

The realities of the current U.S. demographical incidence and projections coupled with the current health care disparities underscore the importance of providing culturally competent health care services. Improving the effectiveness and efficiency of health care to racial and ethnic minorities will ultimately improve care for all patients alike. Implications extend to financial incentives for decreasing the staggering costs of health care. Considerable resources are available and invested in the U.S. system of health care. Not addressing avoidable disparities in health care delivery risks minimizing the returns on investments for economic, individual, and societal levels. The structure of the current U.S. health care system and the fact that there is a gap in the growing racial and ethnic minorities population in relation to minority providers of health care services, in addition to the long-standing disparities in health care, makes cultural competence a necessary mandate for all providers of health care services in any setting. Of importance, accrediting and regulatory bodies as well as governmental and payor organizations now request culturally competent health care services. Health care organizations that embrace and promote culturally competent health services are not only doing the right thing, but they are leading the way toward meeting regulatory and accreditory requirements, which one day will have enormous benefit to the consumer and the overall health care delivery system. Any of the models presented in this chapter, in addition to the tools presented, can support providers to deliver optimal care. Although the fundamental inequalities that exist in society (including social, economic, and environmental factors) are important contextual contributors to health care disparities, health care professionals have both the professional and ethical mandates to deliver care that will result in optimal outcomes for all patients.

Case Scenarios in Long-Term Care

In order to fully understand the value of culturally competent health care, consider the following two clinical case examples and questions for critical thinking and reflection. Group discussion with staff can follow.

Case Study 6.1: Home Health Care Agency

Joy James, a field nurse RN, works for the Carters Home Health Care Agency and supervises the Home Health Aides (HHA). Joy received a complaint from Mrs. Abraham, a Muslim patient, for whom she has been managing pain caused by Multiple Myeloma. Mrs. Abraham informed Joy that she no longer wants the HHA Tammy, because every time Tammy visits her she complains about the need to take off her shoes at the doorstop. She also forgets to replace her pain relief soap under her pillows; this causes her to suffer severe pain until there is someone available to replace the soap under her pillows. Joy asked Tammy about the complaint she received. Tammy stated that Mrs. Abraham is very superstitious and must be confused. Tammy did not replace the soap because she knows it is superstitious, and she does not understand how soap under Mrs. Abraham pillows will relieve her pain. Tammy stated: "I gave her a good back rub with lotion that should help her pain more than a soap under her pillows." Joy concluded, "I am tired of all this, I just have to discharge her, or consult the Psychiatrist."

Useful Critical Thinking Points to Shape Discussions With Nursing Staff for Home Health Care: Case 1

1. What did we note regarding cultural beliefs?

   Recall that cultural beliefs of the client influence the extent to which an individual will accept or reject a recommended treatment. Clinicians must be cognizant of the cultural uniqueness of the client, specifically as it relates to treatment options.

2. What was Tammy trying to do to Mrs. Abraham? What does Tammy need to learn to help her understand patients like Mrs. Abraham?

   As indicated by her behavior, the Home Health Aide Tammy is not sensitive to the cultural beliefs and practices of her patient. It may be helpful for the aide to have a conversation about the cultural specific needs and preferences of the client. Tammy must determine from the client's perception what works or does not work for relief of her pain. Tammy must also respect the wishes of the client with removal of shoes prior to entering the house.

3. Do you think Joy could have handled the situation in a better way?

   In her supervisory role, Joy has the responsibility of providing optimal levels of culturally congruent care for a cadre of patients. She must strive to increase awareness, knowledge, and sensitivity of the cultural health beliefs and practices of all patients, and in this case a Muslim patient. Thus, she must work with the aide in helping her to begin the process of developing knowledge and sensitivity to this client. Referring the client to a psychiatrist when not needed wastes scarce economic resources. Thus, RNs must accurately assesses their patients' cultural health beliefs and design appropriate interventions that will ultimately improve client adherence to treatment and improve and contain cost.

4. What do you think about placing soap under a patient's pillow? Will it relieve her pain or serve as a pain management technique?

   In bridging the clinician–client cultural gap, the clinician must learn about the client's cultural belief (assessment) about the efficacy of soap under a pillow. Such a practice may not exist in Western medicine, or may be interpreted as not having biomedical bearing. The lesson is, however, that clinicians should do their best to accommodate client's requests, especially if accommodating the patient's cultural health beliefs does not place the patient at risk or result in potential harm to the patient. In certain situations, the clinician can use the patient's choice of intervention to complement the Western intervention. If the patient believes that it is helpful to complement conventional therapy, then it is alright to be included as a part of the plan treatment.

5. Give examples of practices you thought were ridiculous that patients have requested you to implement to help with their illness. How did you react then? Will you react differently now?

The journey of becoming a culturally competent provider is a process of developing sensitivity, knowledge, and requisite skill when providing care for those different from you. With frequent clinical encounters, the clinician progresses from being a novice to becoming more proficient in culturally sensitive situations.

6. How do your own personal beliefs contradict with those of the patients?

It is essential for providers to "know thyself" and develop greater awareness about biases, prejudices, and stereotypical ideas of the "other." During the clinical encounter, the clinician must obtain culturally specific information about the client. In some situations, the personal beliefs of the clinician and patient will differ, but this should not be a barrier for providing culturally congruent care.

Useful Critical Thinking Points to Shape Discussions for the Nursing Home: Case 2

1. What do you think of Casey? How can we help her do her job better?

In this situation, the CNA perceives herself as being quite experienced and competent in her practice. She resents the interference and knowledge expertise and lacks respect for

---

Case Study 6.2: The Nursing Home

Casey has been working at Boomers NH as a Certified Nursing Assistant (CNA) for 13 years and knows her duties very well. Anna is the nursing supervisor of the NH and has worked as an RN in several countries. She received her basic nursing education in India and recently emigrated from Ireland. Lisa is the LPN in charge of the 4-west wing of the NH. The patient, Mrs. Yu, newly admitted to the NH because of Cerebral Vascular Accident (CVA) complicated with right-sided paralysis, hails from China. During supervisory rounds, Anna noticed Casey making her best effort to feed Mrs. Yu through the side of the mouth where there is some muscle weakness and paralysis. Mrs. Yu would not eat the food.

Anna yelled, "Casey! Stop! What are you doing?" She then approached Lisa, the charge nurse, and warned her to take responsibility for the safety of her patients by appropriately supervising Casey. Casey intercepted, "I know how to feed patients, and no one needs a lesson on feeding people. You cannot come from another country to run this place." Casey now turned to Lisa stating, "These Indian nurses are trifling!" Lisa stated, "I know why Mrs. Yu is not eating; it is not us . . . it is the Yin-Yang thing. . . . She is waiting for her daughter. She only eats when her daughter brings the food."

---

the professional nurse and her racial, ethnic, and country identities. Lisa, the LPN charge nurse, must confront the Certified Nursing Assistant (CNA) about the clinical issues related to "force feeding" of the stroke patient on the side of the mouth with muscle weakness. It is a teachable moment! This cultural clash of providers provides the opportunity for the unit to schedule cultural sensitivity sessions and address issues of bias and prejudice in the workplace with emphasis on respecting the other and ensuring patient safety. In the long run, if not properly addressed, such stress-provoking situations will negatively influence the quality of care.

2. How would you interpret Casey's comment about Indian nurses? Is this type of comment acceptable? If no, why?

Casey's comment about the Indian nurse supervisor clearly demonstrated that she is prejudiced toward an entire ethnic group of nurse professionals whom she perceives as outsiders and perhaps not knowledgeable and informed about the client population. Such behavior is not acceptable in clinical practice, if not morally reprehensible.

3. Why was Mrs. Yu not eating? Does Lisa give us any lead from her assessment of her patient's cultural behavior? What is the Yin-Yang thing?

It appears as if the patient is more comfortable with the food her daughter brings and perhaps prefers her daughter feeding her. Culturally diverse patient populations may not be familiar with some of the Western food often served in NH. They may also not find Western food appetizing. Additionally, in certain cultures, such as the Chinese culture, illness interpretation is based on a balance between "cold" (yin) and "hot" (yang); imbalance implies a diseased state. Patients who attribute the cause of their illness to too much heat in the body will not eat any food that the culture interprets as hot. This does not literally mean hot or cold as in temperature, it has less to do with the actual temperature or moisture of the food and more to do with its "energy." Examples of yin foods are: bananas, broccoli, grapes, lemon, cabbage, barley, toasted bread, baked tofu, and boiled spinach. Examples of yang foods are: roast beef, smoked fish, garlic, ham, onions, peanut butter, and potatoes. As such, health care providers should assess their patients to understand their unique interpretations of illness in order to design appropriate interventions. Further, health care organizations should have infrastructures and policies that support providers to accurately intervene. In this case, visiting hours could be made flexible to allow the daughter to visit as much as necessary and bring home-cooked foods if the patient is not on a special diet, and if so, educate the family member to that effect. Or, the NH kitchen could serve food that meets the patient's culture.

4. What are some of the practices of Western medicine that may seem ridiculous to culturally diverse patient populations?

In many traditional cultures, health care providers are viewed as the experts having the knowledge, power, and authority to advise and make all health care–related decisions on behalf of their patients. Asking the patient for their input or opinion in making health care decisions may be distressful and seen as ridiculous because it places a burden on the patient and the family who do not have the expertise or background knowledge to make the best possible decision. Other situations that may seem ridiculous to culturally diverse patient populations include asking for advance directives or end-of-life decisions, such as "do not resuscitate," on behalf of their loved ones. Some traditional cultures believe that their end of life has already been determined prior to birth, and they have no control over what is going to happen. Asking this patient or family about advance directives or making "do not resuscitate" decisions could distress and also sound ridiculous. That being said, it is important for health care providers to understand that due to acculturation and individual differences, not all culturally diverse patients will be fatalistic in their thought process. This reiterates the importance of individual patient assessment and care planning!

5. Discuss culturally diverse (traditional) and the biomedical (Western) ways of illness interpretation and causes.

Many traditional patient populations hold different views about the causes and meanings of illness, which is very different from the Western biomedical view. Biomedicine explanatory models of illness focus on abnormalities in the structure and function of body organs and systems. For example, tuberculosis in the lung is explained to be due to Tuberculin bacilli and requires specific antibiotic treatment over a long period of time. Traditional cultures tend to interpret the cause of illness in a much different way. As an example, in some cultures, a healthy body is seen to be in harmony or balance and thus able to resist any disease because the forces or energy of yin and yang (cold and hot) are balanced in the body. Disharmony results in diseases, and this happens when the forces or energy of yin and yang are unbalanced in the body. Another explanation of illness is the "Evil Eye." This is the belief that some people can intentionally or unintentionally bring illness upon you by expressing certain feelings, such as envy, or giving a compliment. The person being envied or complimented stands the risk of getting sick, having bad luck, or even dying. See Table 6.4 for a discussion of assessing geriatric nursing competencies.

6.4	Application of AACN's Geriatric Competencies in Relation to Developing Cultural Competence in Long-Term Care
AACN Competency:	**Goals and critical questions to ask:**
1. Critical Thinking	**Goals:** Recognize one's own and others' attitudes, values, and expectations about aging and their impact on care of older adults and their families; adopt the concept of individualized care as the standard of practice with older adults.
	Examples of some critical questions to ask:
	A. What are your own, the providers', and team members' self-reflection of cultural values and beliefs about aging? What are the providers expectations for older adults from diverse cultures and cultural groups?
	B. How is aging valued among various cultures and cultural groups?
	C. Are the health care organization, its team leaders, and team members culturally competent?
2. Communication	**Goals:** Communicate effectively, respectfully, and compassionately with older adults and their families; recognize the biopsychosocial, functional, and spiritual changes of old age.
	Examples of some critical questions to ask:
	A. Are the health care organization, its staff, and team leaders sensitive, knowledgeable, and skilled in their communication to older adults and their families of diverse cultures?
	1. Is written and verbal communication accessible and available in non-English languages?
	2. Are language interpreters accessible when needed?
	3. Are various cultural languages acknowledged in the health care setting?

(Continued)

	Application of AACN's Geriatric Competencies in Relation to Developing Cultural Competence in Long-Term Care *(Continued)*
6.4	

AACN Competency:	Goals and critical questions to ask:
2. Communication (Continued)	B. Do the health care organization, its staff, and team leaders recognize or take into consideration the impact of sensory age-related changes for culturally diverse groups? C. Are the health care organization, its team leaders, and team members culturally competent?
3. Assessment	<u>Goals</u>: Incorporate into daily practice valid and reliable tools to assess the biopsychosocial, functional, and spiritual status of older adults; assess the living environment with special awareness of the biopsychosocial and functional changes common in old age; analyze the effectiveness of community resources in assisting older adults and their families to maintain independence; assess family knowledge of skills necessary to deliver care to older adult. <u>Examples of some critical questions to ask</u>: A. Do health care organizations, their team leaders, and members utilize assessment tools and techniques for history taking and physical assessment that take into consideration language barriers and knowledge about different cultures? B. Are there existing language or cultural barriers that prohibit effective teaching to family members or patients about their condition and its management? If so, how can this barrier be eliminated?
4. Technical Skill	<u>Goals</u>: Adapt technical skills to meet the functional, biopsychosocial, and endurance capabilities of older adults; individualize care and prevent morbidity and mortality associated with the use of physical and chemical restraints in older adults.

(Continued)

149

AACN Competency:	Goals and critical questions to ask:
4. Technical Skill (Continued)	<u>Examples of some critical questions to ask</u>: A. Are staff culturally sensitive and aware of technical skills that may or may not be culturally acceptable to older adults? B. Has a language or cultural barrier influenced staff's consideration of use of physical or chemical restraints in an older adult? C. How is care individualized for older adults of diverse cultures and languages?
5. Core Knowledge: Health Promotion, Risk Reduction, Disease Prevention	<u>Goals</u>: Prevent or reduce common risk factors that contribute to functional decline, impaired quality of life, excess disability in older adults; follow standards of care to recognize and report elder mistreatment; apply evidence-based standards to reduce risk, screen, immunize, and promote healthy lifestyles in older adults. <u>Examples of some critical questions to ask</u>: A. Does the health care organization, its team leader, or members utilize established national clinical guidelines for the assessment and management of various conditions unique to care of older adults and those of various cultures? (For example, assessment of type 2 diabetes, elder mistreatment, injury prevention, urinary incontinence and polypharmacy?) If not, is there access to these guidelines and documents? B. Does the health care organization, its team leader, or members refer to Healthy People 2010's guidelines for the prevention and management of diseases and conditions affecting older adults?
6. Core Knowledge: Illness and Disease Management	<u>Goals</u>: Recognize and manage geriatric syndromes common to older adults; recognize the complex interaction of acute and chronic comorbidities common to older adults.

(Continued)

AACN Competency:	Goals and critical questions to ask:
6. Core Knowledge: Illness and Disease Management (Continued)	<u>Examples of some critical questions to ask</u>: A. Does the team leader and its members recognize various presentations and the management of geriatric syndromes among older adults of culturally diverse backgrounds? B. Do team members recognize the excess morbidity and mortality associated with diseases as they occur among culturally diverse age-groups?
7. Core Knowledge: Information and Health Care Technology	<u>Goals</u>: Use of technology to enhance older adults' function, independence, and safety; facilitate communication through transitions across and between various care settings. <u>Examples of some critical questions to ask</u>: A. Do the team leader and team members recognize the meaning, value, and beliefs held by older adults who utilize various technologies to improve sensory, communication, or functional impairment, such as eyeglasses, use of hearing aids, canes, walkers, or use of wheelchair and other adaptive devices?
8. Core Knowledge: Ethics	<u>Goals</u>: Assist older adults, families, and caregivers to understand and balance everyday autonomy and safety decisions; apply legal and ethical principles to the complex issues that arise in care of older adults. <u>Examples of some critical questions to ask</u>: A. In the health care organization or community setting, do language or cultural barriers exist that pose threats to the older adults autonomous decision making? Safety? Security or ability to live independently?

(Continued)

6.4

Application of AACN's Geriatric Competencies in Relation to Developing Cultural Competence in Long-Term Care *(Continued)*

AACN Competency:	Goals and critical questions to ask:
9. Core Knowledge: Human Diversity	<u>Goals</u>: Appreciate the influence of attitudes, roles, language, culture, race, religion, gender, and lifestyle on how families and assistive personnel provide long-term care to older adults. <u>Examples of some critical questions to ask</u>: A. Is there a cultural gap between the provider–patient? If so, how is it identified and managed? B. Does the cultural gap between provider–patient influence patient satisfaction with care? C. Does the health care facility take the necessary steps to identify the cultural gaps and to provide for culturally appropriate solutions for effective delivery of health care?
10. Core Knowledge: Global Health Care	<u>Goals</u>: Evaluate differing international models of geriatric care. <u>Examples of some critical questions to ask</u>: A. What types of health care models have older adult residents experienced from various countries and cultures? How has their experience influenced, if at all, their understanding and value of the current model of delivery of health care?
11. Core Knowledge: Health Care Systems	<u>Goals</u>: Analyze the impact of an aging society on the nation's health care system; evaluate the influence of payer systems on access, availability, and affordability of health and policy care. <u>Examples of some critical questions to ask</u>: A. Are the health care services available to the older adult utilized? Are they affordable? Accessible? And are they appropriate for older adults of diverse cultures?

(Continued)

6.4

Application of AACN's Geriatric Competencies in Relation to Developing Cultural Competence in Long-Term Care (*Continued*)

AACN Competency:	Goals and critical questions to ask:
12. Core Knowledge: Provider of Care	<u>Goals:</u> Recognize the benefits of inter-disciplinary teams in care of older adults; evaluate the utility of complementary and integrative health practice on health promotion and symptom management. <u>Examples of some critical questions to ask:</u> A. Do the health care organization, team leaders, and health care providers recognize, utilize, or explore use of complementary and integrative health care practices when caring for older adults of diverse cultures? If not, why not? B. Are structures, policy, and resources available to support culturally competent care in the health care setting?
13. Core Knowledge: Designer/Manager and Coordinator of Care	<u>Goals:</u> Facilitate older adults' active participation in all aspects of their own health care; involve, educate, and include significant others in implementing best practices for older adults; ensure quality of care commensurate with older adults' vulnerability and frequency/intensity of care needs. <u>Critical questions to ask:</u> A. Are there cultural barriers influencing the older adults' participation or education about health care activities?
14. Core Knowledge: Member of a Profession	<u>Goals:</u> Promote quality preventive and end-of-life care for older adults as essential, desirable, and integral components of nursing practice.

(Continued)

6.4	Application of AACN's Geriatric Competencies in Relation to Developing Cultural Competence in Long-Term Care *(Continued)*
AACN Competency:	**Goals and critical questions to ask:**
14. Core Knowledge: Member of a Profession (Continued)	<u>Critical questions to ask:</u> A. What cultural values, beliefs exist for older adults facing end-of-life care decisions? Are these values and beliefs supported within the health care organization? Within the state or territory of care? In accordance to state health policy?

Note: Table developed by D. Gray-Miceli.
Source: American Association of Colleges of Nursing. The John A. Hartford Foundation Institute For Geriatric Nursing. (2000). *Older adults: Recommended baccalaureate competencies and curricular guidelines for geriatric nursing care.* Washington, DC: Author.

References

American Nurses Association (ANA). (1991). *Position statement on cultural diversity in nursing practice.* Washington, DC: Author. Retrieved August 27, 2007, from http://www.nursingworld.org/readroom/position/ethics/etcldv.htm

Anderson, L. M., Scrimshaw, S. C., Fullilove, M. T., Fielding, J. E., & Normand, J. (2003). Culturally competent healthcare systems: A systematic review. *American Journal of Preventive Medicine, 24*(3S), 68–79.

Berlin, E. A., & Fowkes, W. C., Jr. (1983). A teaching framework for cross-cultural health care — Application in family practice, in cross-cultural medicine. *Western Journal of Medicine, 12,* 93–98, 139.

Betancourt, J. R., Green, A. R., & Carrillo, J. E. (2002). *Cultural competence in health care: Emerging framework and practical approaches.* New York: The Commonwealth Fund.

Bigby, J. A. (Ed.). (2003). *Cross-cultural medicine.* Philadelphia, PA: American College of Physicians.

Campinha-Bacote, J. (2002). The process of cultural competence in the delivery of healthcare services: A model of care. *Journal of Transcultural Nursing, 13*(3), 181–184.

Campinha-Bacote, J., Betancourt, J. R., Carrillo, J. E., & Green, A. R. (1999). Hypertension in multicultural and minority populations: Linking communication to compliance. *Current Hypertension Report, 1,* 482–488.

Cooper, L. A., & Powe, N. R. (2004). *Disparities in patient experiences, healthcare processes, and outcomes: The role of patient-provider racial, ethnic, and language concordance.* (Publication 753). New York, NY: The Commonwealth Fund.

Di Clemente, R. J., & Wingwood, G. M. (1995). A randomized controlled trial of an HIV sexual risk reduction intervention for young African-American women. *Journal of the American Medical Association, 16,* 1271–1276.

Giger, J. N., & Davidhizar, R. E. (2004). *Transcultural nursing: Assessment & intervention* (4th ed.). St. Louis, MO: Mosby.

Giger, J., Davidhizar, R. E., Purnell, L., Harden, J. T., Phillips, J., & Strickland, O. (2007). American Academy of Nursing expert panel report: Developing cultural competence to eliminate health disparities in ethnic minorities and other vulnerable populations. *Journal of Transcultural Nursing, 18*(2), 95–102.

Goode, T. D., Dunne, M. C., & Bronheim, S. M. (2006). The evidence base for cultural and linguistic competency in health care. The Commonwealth Fund. Retrieved September 6, 2007, from http://www.commonwealthfund.org/publications/publications_show.htm?doc_id=413821

Institute of Medicine. (2001). *Crossing the quality chasm: A new health system for the 21st century.* Washington, DC: National Academy Press.

Institute of Medicine. (2003). *Unequal treatment: Confronting racial and ethnic disparities in health care.* Washington, DC: National Academy Press.

Institute of Medicine. (2004). *Health literacy: A prescription to end confusion.* Washington, DC: National Academies Press.

Kleinman, A., Eisenberg, L., & Good, B. (1978). Culture, illness, and care: Clinical lessons from anthropologic and cross-cultural research. *Annals of Internal Medicine, 88,* 251–258.

Lavizzo-Mourey, R., & Mackenzie, E. R. (1996). Cultural competence: Essential measurements of quality for managed care organizations. *Annals of Internal Medicine, 124*(10), 919–921.

Leah, S. K., Jacobs, E. A., Chen, A. H., & Sunita, M. (2007). Do professional interpreters improve clinical care for patients with limited English proficiency? *A Systematic Review of the Literature Health Services Research, 42*(2), 727–754.

Leff, J. (1981). Psychiatry around the globe: A transcultural view. NY: Marcel Dekker, Inc.

Leininger, M. M. (2002). Culture care theory: A major contribution to advance transcultural nursing knowledge and practices. *Journal of Trans-Cultural Nursing, 13*(3), 189–192.

Levinson, W., Roter, D. L., Mullooly, J. P., Dull, V. T., & Frankel, R. M. (1997). Physician-patient communication: The relationship with malpractice claims among primary care physicians and surgeons. *Journal of the American Medical Association, 277*(7), 553–559.

Meleis, A. I. (2005). *Theoretical nursing: Development & progress.* Philadelphia: Lippincott, Williams, Wilkins.

Ngo-Metzger, Q., Telfair, D. H., & Sorkin, D. H. (2006). *Cultural competency and quality of care: Obtaining the patient's perspective.* The Commonwealth Fund. Retrieved September 7, 2007, from http://www.commonwealthfund.org/publications/publications_show.htm?doc_id=414116#areaCitation

Purnell, L. (2002). The Purnell model for cultural competence. *Journal of Transcultural Nursing, 13*(3), 193–196.

Spector, R. E. (2004). *Cultural diversity in health & illness* (6th ed.). Upper Saddle River, NJ: Prentice Hall.

U.S. Census Bureau. (2000). Current population survey, Census 2000, the statistical abstract of the United States and the Census Bureau's international database.

U.S. Census Bureau. (2005). *Nation's population one-third minority.* Retrieved May 15, 2005, from http://www.census.gov/PressRelease/www/releases/archives/population/006808.html

U.S. Department of Commerce. Minority Business Development Agency. (1999). *Minority population growth: 1995–2050.* Retrieved September 2, 2007, from http://www.mbda.gov/documents/mbdacolor.pdf

U.S. Department of Health and Human Services. (2001). *National standards for culturally and linguistically appropriate services in health care: Final report.* Office of Minority Health. Retrieved January 22, 2008, from http://www.omhrc.gov/clas/finalcultural1a.htm

U.S. Department of Health and Human Services. (2004) *The registered nurse population: Findings from the 2004 national sample survey of registered nurses.* Washington, DC: Author. Retrieved January 22, 2008, from http://bhpr.hrsa.gov/healthworkforce/rnsurvey04/2.htm

U.S. Department of Health and Human Services. Office of Minority Health. (n.d.). *What is cultural competency.* Retrieved August 28, 2007, from http://www.omhrc.gov/templates/browse.aspx?lvl=2&lvlID=11

Virshup, B., Oppenberg, A., & Coleman, M. (1999). Strategic risk management: Reducing malpractice claims through more effective patient-doctor communication. *American Journal of Medical Quality, 14*(4), 153–159.

Wynia, M., & Matiasek, J. (2006). *Promising practices for patient-centered communication with vulnerable populations: Examples from eight hospitals.* The Commonwealth Fund. Retrieved September 7, 2007, from http://www.commonwealthfund.org/publications/publications_show.htm?doc_id=397067

Developing Cultural Competence in Long-Term Care Nursing
Post-test (circle one)

Please circle the *best* answer among the items listed below.

1. Culturally competent care is best defined as:

   a. The use of one's personal experience to treat patients and staff.

   b. Using the institution's cultural staff to meet the needs of the patients and other staff.

   c. Understanding another culture that is different from one's own culture and using that knowledge to treat everyone else the same way.

   d. A set of skills, knowledge, and attitudes that respect the values of others when rendering care, even when it conflicts with one's own personal beliefs or values.

2. Health care organizations need to provide culturally competent care because:

   a. It is documented in the Constitution of the United States.

   b. Many people cannot speak English or have limited proficiency in English.

   c. Of changing demographics, reports of health disparities, current legislative protocols, and evidence of positive patient outcomes.

   d. Organizations will be able to receive more money from the government.

3. Cultural sensitivity is best described as:

   a. Being sensitive and respectful of the values and beliefs of others, which may or may not conflict one's own values and beliefs.

   b. Knowing that cultural differences and similarities exist within and between groups without assigning value to the differences.

c. A process of changing one's personal values to those of others.

d. Trying to learn another language so one can help the patients.

4. What is the first step to becoming a culturally competent health care provider?

   a. Talking with someone from another culture all the time.
   b. Self-appraisal of one's own cultural values and beliefs.
   c. Listening and learning languages other than English.
   d. Taking classes to learn all the possible cultures in the world.

5. Choose the five strategies for bridging the cultural health gap, as outlined by Berlin and Fowkes?

   a. Assess, Explain, Evaluate, Implement, and Observe (AEEIO)
   b. Explain, Negotiate, Decide, Overcome, and Sign (ENDOS)
   c. Listen, Explain, Acknowledge, Recommend, and Negotiate (LEARN)
   d. Assess, Decide, Implement, Evaluate, and Report (ADIER)

6. Which one of the following would not be an effective strategy for cross-cultural communication?

   a. Having respect for the values of others
   b. Seeing differences in others as primarily weaknesses
   c. Seeing differences as strengths rather than weaknesses
   d. Recognizing unfamiliar situations as interesting instead of annoying

7. Communication about health beliefs and practices of residents/patients requires that culturally competent providers:

   a. Discuss the meaning of health and illness, its etiology, and cultural-specific concerns.
   b. Provide opportunity for patients to describe their symptoms and approaches for coping with stressors.
   c. Discuss the role of the family during sickness.
   d. All of the above

Match the following terms on the *left* to the correct definitions on the *right*.

Term		Definition

Term

  8. **Ethnicity** _____

  9. **Stereotype** _____

10. **Racism** _____

11. **Discrimination** _____

12. **Cultural knowledge** _____

Definition

A. Belief that race is the primary determinant of human traits and capabilities and the inherent superiority of a particular race.

B. Intentional or unintentional actions against a group or individuals based on gender, racial groups, ethnicity, sexual orientation, or education.

C. Self-defined affiliation with a specific group or subgroup that shares common cultural heritage due to history, customs, and language passed on from generation to generation.

D. A fixed picture or set mental image that is used to represent all people from a group.

E. Familiarization with cultural history, values, and belief systems of the members of another group.

Participant Evaluation Form
Developing Cultural Competence in Long-Term Care Nursing

Today's Date ___/___/___   Facility: _____

Please circle the best response.

Example: Strongly Disagree   Disagree   Agree   Strongly Agree
                     1   2   3   4

At the end of the presentation I can:

1. Discuss the importance of cultural competence health care services

Strongly Disagree   Disagree   Agree   Strongly Agree
         1   2   3   4

2. Discuss strategies for effective cross-cultural communication

Strongly Disagree   Disagree   Agree   Strongly Agree
         1   2   3   4

3. Discuss some health beliefs and practices of diverse cultural groups

Strongly Disagree   Disagree   Agree   Strongly Agree
         1   2   3   4

4. Be more aware of my own cultural values and beliefs

Strongly Disagree   Disagree   Agree   Strongly Agree
         1   2   3   4

5. Discuss legislative and regulatory mandates about cultural competence

Strongly Disagree   Disagree   Agree   Strongly Agree
         1   2   3   4

6. Discuss strategies to bridge cultural gaps

Strongly Disagree   Disagree   Agree   Strongly Agree
         1   2   3   4

7. Identify some of the barriers to providing cultural competent care

Strongly Disagree	Disagree	Agree	Strongly Agree
1	2	3	4

8. This program will help me work better with the clients/ patients

Strongly Disagree	Disagree	Agree	Strongly Agree
1	2	3	4

9. This program will help me work better with other staff

Strongly Disagree	Disagree	Agree	Strongly Agree
1	2	3	4

Overall, I rate:

10. This program

Poor	Fair	Good	Excellent
1	2	3	4

11. The case studies

Poor	Fair	Good	Excellent
1	2	3	4

12. Speaker 1 _____ [insert name]

Poor	Fair	Good	Excellent
1	2	3	4

13. Speaker 2 _____ [insert name]

Poor	Fair	Good	Excellent
1	2	3	4

14. This program would be better if:

15. What other cultural competence topics would be helpful to you in the future?

Your ID _____   RN _____ Non RN _____
Today's Date ____/____/____   Facility: _____

Leading Through Education in Long-Term Care Nursing

Pre-test (circle one)

1. Name two characteristics of adult learners.

    a.   _____

    b.   _____

Please circle the *best* answer among the items listed below.

Example:

This is a test.

   a.   No, this is not a test.
   ⓑ   Yes, this is a test.
   c.   No, this is a joke.

The answer is ⓑ so it will be circled.

2. The education development process consists of:

    a.   Needs assessment, objectives, design, and evaluation
    b.   Needs assessment, teaching, reinforcement, and feedback
    c.   Planning, delivery, and evaluation
    d.   Planning, teaching objectives, delivery, and evaluation

3. Objectives are behavioral when they:

    a.   Address behavior on the job
    b.   Identify what the teacher will do
    c.   Target what learners will be able to do
    d.   Specify the domain of learning addressed

4. Needs assessment data appropriately include: (circle all that apply)

    a.   Identified competencies/job description
    b.   Focus groups
    c.   Survey data
    d.   Organization policies

e. Course outlines from professional meetings
f. Supervisor observations/reports
g. Quality Improvement data

5. Assumptions about adult learners include: (circle all that apply)

   a. Self-concept
   b. Experience
   c. Job level/position
   d. Readiness
   e. Motivation

6. The domains of learning include:

   a. Motivation, readiness, and self-concept
   b. Attitude, self-concept, and experience
   c. Skill, attitude, and readiness
   d. Knowledge, skill, and attitude

7. Teaching and learning experiences that might involve modifying a learner's attitudes include: (circle all that apply)

   a. Experiential or reflective
   b. Role play
   c. Crossword puzzles
   d. Perception exercise
   e. Exposing myths and stereotypes
   f. Demonstration

8. An example of an objective that involves learners mastering new information (knowledge) is:

   a. Manage personal feelings while caring for persons with dementia.
   b. Use a range of assessment strategies to identify the meaning of behavior.
   c. Individualize care to older adults with dementia to prevent and respond to behaviors.
   d. Discuss behavior as a form of communication.

9. Formative evaluation: (circle all that apply)

   a. Is when the cook tastes the soup.
   b. Sums up the program (person) with the aim of making decisions.
   c. Takes place while the program (person) is being formed with the aim of improvement.
   d. Is when the guests taste the soup.

10. The four levels of evaluation get progressively more challenging. Level 1: Reaction, measures the following:

    a. The impact of the educational program in relation to organizational needs and goals
    b. The ability of the learner to demonstrate acquisition of the knowledge, skills, or attitudinal objectives at the time of the program
    c. The ability of the learner to perform the cognitive, skill, and other objectives in the work
    d. How the learner felt about the program, how it met needs, and opinions about components of the program

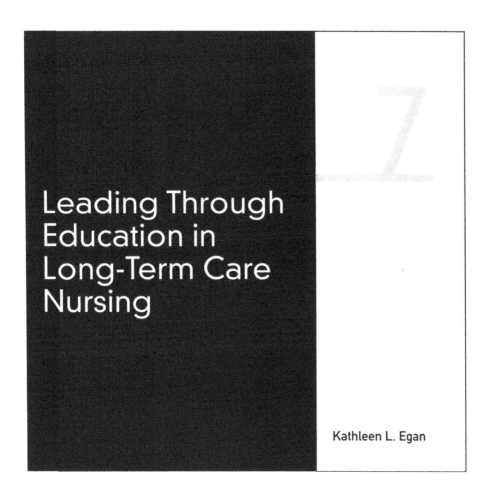

Leading Through Education in Long-Term Care Nursing

Kathleen L. Egan

Registered nurses (RNs) in the expanding range of long-term care settings demonstrate their leadership by educating other nursing and direct care staff. Yet, when confronted with the need to develop an education program, nurses often realize that their own experience as learners is their primary preparation for this role. Few have received formal education as educators. This chapter is intended to provide the nurse with a framework for developing education for adult learners in long-term care. One might ask, "Why not simply pick up a general text on nursing education?" Some of the major reasons for this chapter are listed here. In short, there are challenges particular to the long-term care environment and to the learners found in those settings that will not be found in the pages of a general text on nursing education. Consider the interplay of these reasons in the context of the workplace:

- *Resources for on-the-job education in long-term care are typically limited.* Frequently there is little or no budget support for program development, faculty, or educational technology, and staff shortages and overload are common, making it difficult to release staff for education time. Even when staff members can attend, the time available is limited, often to an hour, half-hour, or even less. This significantly limits the amount and depth of content that can be covered. Staff barely have the time to transition into a learning mode and may be preoccupied with the work left behind or yet to be completed.

- *It can be difficult to motivate and interest learners.* There are many reasons why direct care staff may not be responsive to invitations to in-service education, such as external requirements, prior negative experiences with education, and their own perceptions of what they need, which may be different from the instructor's. Staff members come to the work environment with preconceived ideas and beliefs about health care, patient care, and education. Their level of education achieved may also influence the value or importance placed on educational programs in the workplace.

- *The environment is highly regulated.* In many settings, the in-service education programs required each year, such as fire safety or infection control, become repetitive, and nurses are challenged to find interesting and innovative ways to present the material differently each year so as to stimulate the learner. In addition, regulation dictates staff functions and leaves little time or opportunity for learning for its own sake.

Staff members come to the work environment with preconceived ideas and beliefs about health care, patient care, and education. Their level of education achieved may also influence the value or importance placed on educational programs in the workplace.

These reasons all substantiate the assertion that staff education in long-term care and other practice settings is a challenging and complex role to execute effectively. RN staff members providing education effectively and efficiently have learned important strategies to overcome the competition between two very important deliverables: providing quality patient care and educating staff about how to provide quality patient care.

Within this context, nurses who care for older adults by providing quality patient care utilize many of the essential geriatric competencies outlined by the American Association of Colleges of Nursing (AACN) in their document *The Essentials of Baccalaureate Education for Professional Nursing Practice.* Relative to AACN's document, we recognize that this teaching and learning module integrates all of the 14 core competencies outlined. In particular, effective educational modules utilize and promote critical thinking among educators and learners; effective communication; state-of-the-science knowledge related to assessment, technical skills, health promotion, and disease prevention; illness and disease management; information and health care technology; ethics and human diversity; global health care; health care systems and policy; and issues germane to providers of care.

Purpose

The intent of this chapter is to give you some tools for planning and delivering education whether it is through in-service education, orientation, giving a presentation, or coaching/mentoring another staff member. It is also intended that this module be useful across a variety of sites where care is delivered—nursing homes, PACE (Programs for All-Inclusive Care of the Elderly), home care, day care, and similar settings. Increasingly, long-term care is moving into community practice settings, and staff training needs to be responsive and adaptable to an increasing range of environments. The principles of sound staff education are the same, irrespective of the practice setting, and are general enough to be useful across settings. So let's take a look at what will help the most as you begin planning an educational program.

What Should You Be Able to Do at the End of This Chapter?

There will still be much left to your creativity, but at the end of this module you should be better able to:

1. Describe a process for developing staff education programs;
2. Describe the principles of adult education and their application to staff development;
3. Describe the domains of learning and the levels of evaluation; and
4. Identify strategies to apply the model, principles, and domains of learning into the long-term care setting.

Let us look at a common scenario in staff development. You are asked to develop an in-service education program on falls and their prevention. This request comes after several elders in your program's care have fallen, and the quality improvement (QI) committee is looking into factors associated with the falls. So, a common clinical problem, for instance fall prevention, is to be taught, but there is no formal content developed and little staff interest. You do not have good educational materials at hand, and you have no budget or outside expert to call. Furthermore, staff members at your facility seem to dislike in-service education programs, and it is difficult to attract staff to participate. How do you address these seemingly insurmountable barriers to creating a successful fall prevention education program?

Where Do You Start?

Critically *think* for a moment, and list the thoughts and questions that initially come to you as you anticipate developing this education program. Your list might include any of the following or a number of others:

- How is fall prevention accomplished at your program?
- What do staff members know about falls? Critically ask yourself, how do I know or measure the staff's current knowledge? Who else may need education about falls and prevention, for example, patients and caregivers?
- Do staff members perceive the need for more education on falls?
- What will result in less frequent falls? Is there any new literature or evidence-based practice for falls prevention that must be included in order to provide quality patient care?
- Where and when can education be scheduled so it is convenient for staff to attend?
- What can you do to make it interesting? Critically *think:* How can the program appeal to a diverse audience who learn by different mechanisms? If I choose to incorporate interactive learning strategies, what do I choose, and how do I choose this?
- Who will teach it? Critically *think:* Should the adult learner audience be mixed from various disciplines, for instance, should I include the dietary departments or physical therapy and various levels of nursing staff (licensed and unlicensed staff)?

Education Development Process

It can be difficult to know where to start. How can you sort through the issues, gather information you need and develop a plan of action that's going to be effective? Consider the following Education Development Process as a mechanism to give you a logical framework for designing any education program, including staff development.

Figure 7.1 shows the elements of the education development process.

Needs Assessment: The First Step

The first and critical step in developing an education program is to identify the education needs of your learners. Like many nursing processes, the education process begins with assessment, in this case, of your learners. Educational needs assessment can be defined as a systematic process for identifying the gap between learners' existing knowledge, skills, and attitudes and the needed knowledge, skills, and attitudes. In staff development, we might add "to do their work effectively." How do you go about such an assessment, especially when time is limited? What are the sources you can use for identifying the needs of your learners? You might start with the following list:

- Required competencies (job description) for your setting
- In our example of an in-service education on falls, you might look at the roles of various staff in fall prevention, assessment, and post-fall review. Do various levels of staff

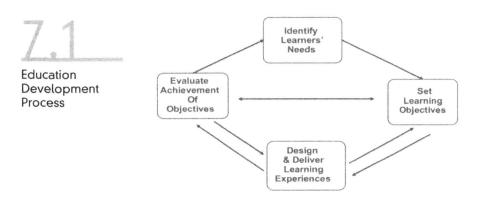

7.1

Education
Development
Process

perform distinctly different aspects of the role, and if so, what are the educational needs based on these roles?

- Quality data or improvement projects
  As staff gather data on the fall history at your program, the QI committee may help you to identify where education is needed, for example, documenting the circumstances of the fall that have occurred or gaps in practice or knowledge. Analysis of the fall reports on the unit may reveal that environmental factors are the cause of a fall, thus requiring further focused educational programs in this particular area.
- Supervisor or team observations and reports
  Conversations with supervisors or team members may be helpful in interpreting or supplementing QI data. In this case, effective communication skills can reveal important areas that continue to surface in review of fall events, such as that performed by facilities that perform a root-causes analysis.
- Learners' self-assessment
  Likewise, conversations with or surveys of your target audience can suggest where they feel education would help most.
- Learners' characteristics
  What do you know about your learners' interests, ambitions, reading levels, educational history, or learning styles? Any of these can help you to design effective education.
- Literature and research, including adult education
  If you have access to the Internet, multiple resources are available online. Otherwise, you may need to seek out an advanced practice nurse or administrator with access to journals and guidelines from national organizations.
  You probably don't have time to tap all of these sources for every in-service, but the more of them you use overtime, the better framework you will have for your work. As a general rule, however, do use more than one source so that you have an appropriate balance in your needs assessment. Multiple sources usually give you the most reliable indicators of needs.

Table 7.1 is an outline of helpful resources starting with the learners and progressing through facility administrators, agency personnel, and professional sources. Consider all of these sources and methods as you complete the First Step: Needs Assessment. As a practice exercise, it is also wise to critically analyze your own learning needs, style, and approaches to teaching. For instance, consider the following exercise.

7.1	Sources and Methods
Learners	Interviews, surveys, suggestion box, focus group
Supervisors, others in contact with learners	Interviews, reports, HR, surveys, focus group, information discussion
Facility/agency	Quality improvement, annual plan, management needs
Professional sources	Review literature on long-term care, nursing, reports on workforce

Exercise: What are your learning needs? Ask yourself: Where are your challenges as an educator? What knowledge or skill do you hope to gain for this module?

Some staff development nurses have identified the need for approaches to deal with learners who are variously described as being fearful of tests, anxious about being "back in school," resentful of being taught, and resistant to change. Of course, some direct care staff are open to education and eager to learn, but those who are described by the list above create a genuine challenge. Let us look to the principles of adult education as a tool for thinking about this learner population.

Adult Education and Andragogy. When they were first articulated in the 1960s and '70s, the principles of adult education shed new light on the ways in which learning is different for adults as compared with children. Adult education was described as *andragogy,* or the "art and science of helping adults learn" (Knowles, 1968), as opposed to *pedagogy,* or the teaching of children. Adult education as a distinct approach makes several assumptions about adult learners:

> *Self-concept:* Adults, as they mature, move from the dependency of childhood to self-direction.
> *Experience:* Over time individuals accumulate an increasing reservoir of experiences that are valuable resources.

Readiness: Adults are ready to learn when real-life tasks or problems require new skills and knowledge.

Problem centered: Adults want to be able to apply what they learn immediately and in real-life situations.

Motivation: As a person matures, the motivation for learning becomes more internal.

Adult education was described as *andragogy,* or the "art and science of helping adults learn" (Knowles, 1968), as opposed to *pedagogy,* or the teaching of children.

These assumptions about adult learners help guide us to develop education that is centered more on the learners than on the content, and to frame it in a way that shows its relevance to their roles and immediate problems, for instance, when taking their experience into account. Individual learners may not live up to all of these assumptions, however. We all know of adults who are very dependent on others for direction, or whose experiences seem to be barriers rather than facilitators of learning. Further, mandated or required education does not fit well with the self-direction of adults or the internal versus external motivation. The challenge is to shape education programs so they serve the individual as well as organizational needs.

The Pennsylvania Intra-Governmental Council on Long-Term Care (2001) surveyed long-term care workers from a variety of settings in Pennsylvania. Table 7.2 reflects what they offered when asked what is important to them in in-service education.

7.2 "In Their Own Words" 2001

Use dedicated trainers who want to train	Use a "buddy" system
Provide more time	Ensure there is a long-term coach
Develop more realistic training	Provide consistency in setting and trainer
First watch, understand, then do	Provide feedback

Key in on understanding residents and clients

Do you see any of the assumptions about adult learners reflected here? What do your trainees tell you are important to them?

In summary, the process of needs assessment identifies the gaps in knowledge, skills, and attitudes by ideally using multiple sources of information and considering the assumptions about adult learners.

Setting Learning Objectives: The Second Step

With at least a preliminary understanding of your learners' needs in hand, you are ready to plan for the outcomes of your education program. Rather than statements of what teachers intend to do (inputs), learning objectives are best set as statements of what learners will be able to do (outcomes). This is because what the learner can do as a result of the education is a better test of the education than what the teacher does. As much as possible, the objectives should describe behaviors and be measurable, which makes them valuable for evaluation of your learners' progress and your program's effectiveness (see Figure 7.1). Let us look at an example of how some identified needs lead to behavioral objectives. Assume you have identified the needs in Table 7.3 and think about whether the objectives meet the criteria of being behavioral and measurable.

The objectives are stated in terms of behaviors, that is, what the participants will be able to do, such as describe or name. They could readily be measured in a pre- post-test assessment.

7.3 Needs and Learning Objectives

Needs	Learning Objectives: "Participants will be able to . . ."
Staff need to understand the progression of dementia	Accurately describe the stages of dementia
Staff need to deal better with challenging behaviors associated with dementia	Name appropriate and inappropriate responses to specific behaviors

Domains of Learning. When developing your objectives, it is useful to consider the three major domains of learning—knowledge, skill, and attitude—and whether you need objectives in each of them (Bloom, 1956, pp. 201–207). Knowledge is almost always important, but will it be enough for learners to "know that" something is true (e.g., after any fall there should be an assessment)? Such knowledge will be relatively useless if they do not "know how" to request or to perform an assessment. Are you confident that staff members accept the importance of a post-fall assessment? Identifying objectives by these domains is also helpful because each learning domain requires different types of learning activities, which in turn require different teaching strategies and resources. When setting your objectives, it is also useful to have in mind the resources available to meet those objectives. Following are examples, continuing to use our falls prevention issue as the focus. Objectives might look like the following:

> *Knowledge:* The learner will be able to describe five interventions that nursing can do to prevent falls.
> *Skill:* The learner will be able to demonstrate a proper foot examination or gait assessment.
> *Attitude:* The learner will show appreciation for the impact of a fall on the older person's confidence in walking.

In summary, your objectives should be based on identified needs, focused on outcomes rather than inputs, reflect behaviors, shaped by the available resources, and keyed to the domains of learning: knowledge, skill, and attitude.

Teaching and Learning Experiences: The Third Step

The needs and the objectives you have identified then guide the learning activities you plan (see Figure 7.1). There are typically multiple approaches to effective teaching and learning of information, skill, and attitude, and which approach you choose may be dictated by your learners, your objectives, your teachers, or other environmental factors, such as the time available, the layout of space and seating (lecture, classroom, round table), and so forth.

Opening and closing the in-service or workshops are important elements as well. If a group of individuals do not know each other, a quick introduction in the form of an icebreaker can help to set the climate you want. If there is not much time, a simple question of "What's your favorite color and why?" can work well. Having individuals introduce themselves to each other in pairs and then to the whole group can be an effective way of helping people feel connected, reduce anxiety, and engage your learners.

In terms of content, a pre-test and a review of learning objectives will orient learners to the focus of the session.

Table 7.4 sorts various learning activities in relation to the domains of learning discussed earlier.

In the knowledge domain, lecture can be a very efficient way of presenting information. Because people often retain only a small proportion of what they hear, it helps to outline what you are going to cover at the beginning, present the information and then review what you have said, pausing to ask or receive questions and verify if your audience is following the content. If you provide *readings* in advance of a program, they orient the learners, raise questions in their minds, and prime them for the learning to come. Assigning reading after the program as a reference can reinforce what has been taught. *Games* can make old content seem newer and introduce an element of fun, and case examples provide a context for information while brainstorming ideas stimulates the audience. Beginning the session with a knowledge quiz or other validated instrument can help to reinforce important points to the learner while also offering an interactive medium

7.4 Teaching and Learning Experiences		
Knowledge	**Skill**	**Attitude**
Lecture reading (text, articles)	Demonstration (positive or negative)	Experiential or reflective
Games	Feedback practice again	Role play
• "Jeopardy/Geropardy"	Case studies	Perception exercise
• Crossword case studies	Brainstorming	Simulations
• Brainstorming		Case studies
		Brainstorming

for presenting content to a learning group who actually work together in health care.

In the skill domain, the key learning experiences are: (1) seeing a skill *demonstrated* correctly, (2) having the opportunity to *practice* the skill, and (3) receiving *feedback* and repeating practice and feedback until the learner can demonstrate the skill. It can be useful to demonstrate the wrong way to perform a skill, especially when that wrong way is common and easily recognized, but then it is important to demonstrate the skill correctly and point out the differences and reasons why one is correct and the other is not.

Simulations can be excellent ways of demonstrating and practicing complex skills such as doing a full assessment of a patient after a fall. Courses teaching CPR use a lot of simulation with models. The opportunity to practice such skills in a setting where patients cannot be harmed is clearly a must. For these patient safety reasons and others, staff may learn using peer-exemplars for learning.

In the domain of attitude, experiential exercises that involve self-reflection are critical. Role play, especially taking roles different from one's own, can provide the opportunity for reflection from a new view point. Often a change in perspective is what is needed to surface and consider one's attitude. Direct care staff may be familiar with exercises that simulate the experience of sensory and other losses in aging. Also, the use of graphics that can be seen in more than one way are helpful to illustrate the possibility of varying perspectives on a given reality. Video clips illustrating scenarios in which attitudes play an important role can also be useful (Delaware Valley Geriatric Education Center of the University of Pennsylvania, 2008). When this is done within a group context, a skilled facilitator should lead the exercise (see Figure 7.1).

In summary, develop teaching and learning experiences that address the objectives and the learning domain of knowledge, skill, or attitude.

Evaluate Achievement of Objectives: The Fourth Step

Nearly everyone involved in an educational program is interested in its evaluation. These include at least those who provided the resources, those involved in planning and teaching the program, and the learners themselves. At the start, it is useful to think of two types of evaluation: learner evaluation and program evaluation. Individual learners are interested in measures of their own success, which may be shown by pre- and post-test scores on a paper and pencil test or by skill demonstration. Improved confidence in their skill and knowledge is also a positive outcome.

The evaluation of the program is, in part, a grouping of individual responses to the program. It asks whether, *on average,* learners gained in knowledge, skill, and attitudinal response (see Table 7.5). Among other important measures are:

- Learner satisfaction
- Improved performance on the job
- Improved job satisfaction

Program evaluation can be thought of as having four increasingly rigorous measures:

Level 1: Reaction—measures how the learner felt about the program, how it met needs, opinions about components of the program

Level 2: Learning—measures the ability of the learner to demonstrate acquisition of the knowledge, skills, or attitudinal objectives at the time of the program

Level 3: Behavior—measures the ability of the learner to perform the cognitive, skill, and other objectives in the work setting

Level 4: Impact—measures the impact of the educational program in relation to organizational needs and goals

7.5 Evaluation: Learner or Program

How well did individual learners meet the objectives?
- Pre/post-test scores (paper or demonstration)
- Improved confidence in role

How well did the program meet its objectives?
- Average or overall gains in knowledge, skill, and attitude
- Learner satisfaction
- Improved performance on the job
- Improved job satisfaction

The evaluation of the program is, in part, a grouping of individual responses to the program. It asks whether, *on average*, learners gained in knowledge, skill, and attitudinal response.

Some of the evaluation methods used at the different levels are reflected in Table 7.6.

In summary, evaluation in the context of an education program can be focused at the level of the learner or the program as a whole. There are multiple levels of program evaluation that can be summarized as measures of reaction to the program, learning of participants, improved behavior or performance on the job, and impact on clients or the clinical setting as a whole. (See Table 7.7.)

Conclusion

In long-term care of the elderly, programs and facilities often turn to education as a remedy for problems in quality of care as well as a recruitment and retention approach to staffing. The RN in long-term care can provide leadership through education by using a systematic process for identifying learning needs, setting objectives, designing learning interventions, and evaluating the program. Careful planning can be used to advocate for greater resources for education with the likelihood of improved outcomes. When comparing the pre-analysis with the post-analysis of the educational program, with positive results (i.e. knowledge and skill improved and possibly attitude changes), then there is increased likelihood that the educational program will be received positively so that staff and patient care will benefit.

Effective teaching and learning promotes the 14 essential competencies for providing quality care to older adults in long-term care. While the educational program in itself should foster

7.6 Evaluation Methods	
Reaction	Questionnaire, interview
Learning	Pre/post-test
Behavior	Follow-up with Trainee or Supervisor; chart review
Impact	Improved care, reduced problems (Quality Improvement/Minimum Data Set)

critical thinking and improved communication as well as state-of-the-science knowledge about health care, education also provides a wonderful forum for teaching about ethics, human diversity, cultural issues, information and technological advances that impact within the health care system, and ultimately shape policy considerations in the global health care arena.

Now, it is time to ask whether the objectives of this chapter were met for you. Are you now able to:

- Describe a process for developing staff education programs?
- Describe the principles of adult education and their application to staff development?
- Describe the domains of learning and the levels of evaluation?
- Identify strategies to apply the model, principles, and domains of learning into the long-term care setting?

7.7 Application of AACN's Geriatric Competencies to Assist in Effective Teaching and Learning in Long-Term Care

AACN Competency:	Goals and critical questions to ask:
1. Critical thinking	Goals: Recognize one's own and others attitudes, values, and expectations about aging and their impact on care of older adults and their families; adopt the concept of individualized care as the standard of practice with older adults.
	Examples of some critical questions to ask:
	A. Does the health care organization participate or promote its health care management team to participate in educational initiatives directed at care of the older adult? For example, are guest lectures invited to conduct educational in-services or are staff members encouraged to attend local educational conferences? How is that knowledge disseminated and shared with other team members?

(Continued)

AACN Competency:	Goals and critical questions to ask:
1. Critical thinking (Continued)	B. How do team members respond to educational in-services about aging? Has the educational intervention been successful in that preconceived views have changed? C. Do team leaders and members acknowledge the value of educational in-services directed at care of the older adult? Does the organization provide for release time to participate in educational interventions off-site?

2. Communication	<u>Goals:</u> Communicate effectively, respectfully, and compassionately with older adults and their families; recognize the biopsychosocial, functional and spiritual changes of old age.
	
	<u>Examples of some critical questions to ask:</u>
	
	A. Do educational materials provide health care staff with written guidelines for communicating effectively, respectfully and compassionately with older adults and their families?
	B. Are educational materials patient-centered? Age-appropriate?
	C. Do educational materials recognize the biopsychosocial, functional and spiritual changes of old age?
	D. Does the team communicate directly with the older adult or family caregiver, if so, are age-appropriate teaching methods incorporated?
	    1. *What are the methods of communication?* Is communication verbal or are written instructions in large bold print provided?
	    2. *Does the team acknowledge each older adult's style of learning or readiness for behavioral change?*

(Continued)

AACN Competency:	Goals and critical questions to ask:
2. Communication (Continued)	3. *Is the speed of delivery of the message altered for older adults with cognitive or sensory impairment?* 4. *Are team recommendations tailored to the older adult who might experience sensory deficits such as visual or hearing loss? (for example, reduction of background noise due to presbycusis; use of large and bold printed materials for visual impairment)* 5. *How is communication delivered to the older adult with transitory stages of cognitive impairment due to delirium or for those with dementia?* 6. *Is adequate time allotted for older adult's feedback & discussion?*

3. Assessment	Goals: Incorporate into daily practice use of valid and reliable tools to assess biopsychosocial, functional and spiritual status; assess the older adults living environment with special awareness of their biopsychosocial and functional status; analyze community resource effectiveness for maintaining functional independence; assess family knowledge of skills needed to deliver care to older adults.
	
	Examples of some critical questions to ask:
	
	A. Is the team performing a clinical assessment of the older adult?
	    1. *If so, what do they know about standard empirically tested measures of geriatric health, function, cognition, psychological, social function? Has their knowledge about these issues been measured?*
	    2. *Do staff feel they need more education on these topics?*

(Continued)

183

AACN Competency:	Goals and critical questions to ask:
4. Technical Skill	<u>Goals:</u> Adapt technical skills to meet the functional, biopsychocosial and endurance capabilities of older adults; individualize care and prevent morbidity and mortality associated with the use of physical and chemical restraints in older adults. A. Do team leaders and staff possess knowledge and technical skill that is age-appropriate? For instance, are they aware of the age-related factors influencing the assessment and presentation of vital signs? Of physical assessment findings? *If not, are there educators available to teach this content and how can they make it interesting?* B. Do team leaders and staff possess knowledge of the harmful effects of physical or chemical restrains in an older adult? Can they identify appropriate behavioral intervention without use of physical or chemical restraint? *If not, are there educators available to teach this content and how can they make it interesting?* C. Is care individualized for older adults within the health care organization? If so, how is this measured? *If not, are there educators available to teach this content and how can they make it interesting?*
5. Core Knowledge: Health Promotion, Risk Reduction	<u>Goals:</u> Prevent or reduce common risk factors that contribute to functional decline, impaired disease prevention quality of life, excess disability in older adults; follow standards of care to recognize and report elder mistreatment; apply evidenced-based standards to reduce risk, screen, immunize and promote healthy lifestyles in older adults. <u>Examples of some critical questions to ask:</u> A. Are educational in-services and educational media available to health care

184

7.7

Application of AACN's Geriatric Competencies to Assist in Effective Teaching and Learning in Long-Term Care (*Continued*)

AACN Competency:	Goals and critical questions to ask:
5. Core Knowledge: Health Promotion, Risk Reduction (Continued)	that identify risk factors for functional decline, geriatric syndromes (for instance, urinary incontinence, falls and pressure sores?) polypharmacy or elder abuse? Are plans of care individualized with current state of the science knowledge and clinical protocols to manage these conditions?
6. Core Knowledge: Illness and Disease Management	<u>Goals:</u> Recognize and manage geriatric syndromes common to older adults; recognize the complex interaction of acute and chronic comorbidities common to older adults. <u>Examples of some critical questions to ask:</u> A. Do health care providers know about and utilize national recommendations and/or clinical practice guidelines in their assessment and management of various health conditions effecting older adults? What are the learner needs in reference to this?
7. Core Knowledge: Information and Health Care Technology	<u>Goals:</u> Use of technology to enhance older adults function, independence and safety; facilitate communication through transitions across and between various care settings. <u>Examples of some critical questions to ask:</u> A. Does the health care organization, its team leaders and members promote and receive regular in-service educational programs on the safety issues related to use of adaptive aides to improve mobility, prevent contractures, pressure sores or sensory impairment? *-Are these adaptive aides current or state of the art technology?* *-Are there efforts to identify learner needs?*
8. Core Knowledge: Ethics	<u>Goals:</u> Assist older adults, families and caregivers to understand and balance 'everyday' autonomy and safety decisions;

(Continued)

7.7

Application of AACN's Geriatric Competencies to Assist in Effective Teaching and Learning in Long-Term Care (*Continued*)

AACN Competency:	Goals and critical questions to ask:
8. Core Knowledge: Ethics (Continued)	apply legal and ethical principles to the complex issues that arise in care of older adults. Examples of some critical questions to ask: A. Do team members possess knowledge about the differences between maintaining autonomy and independence in daily living for old adults? Have you conducted interviews or surveys to ascertain their knowledge, values, and beliefs? B. Does the health care organization perform quality improvement interventions relative to safety?
9. Core Knowledge: Human Diversity	Goals: Appreciate the influence of attitudes, roles, language, culture, race, religion, gender, and lifestyle on how families and assistive personnel provide long-term care to older adults. Examples of some critical questions to ask: A. Does the health care organization and its team leaders provide for educational in-services on human diversity for health care staff? If so, how are learner needs recognized and measured?
10. Core Knowledge: Global Health Care	Goals: Evaluate differing international models of geriatric care. Example of a critical question to ask: A. Does the health care organization educate its staff about the early recognition of older adults who could be transitioned to less dependent situations?
11. Core Knowledge Health Care Systems and Policy	Goals: Analyze the impact of an aging society on the nation's health care system; evaluate the influence of payer systems on access, availability and affordability of health care.

(*Continued*)

7.7

Application of AACN's Geriatric Competencies to Assist in Effective Teaching and Learning in Long-Term Care (*Continued*)

AACN Competency:	Goals and critical questions to ask:
11. Core Knowledge Health Care Systems Policy (Continued)	<u>Example of a critical question to ask:</u> A. Are team members knowledgeable of health care resources for the older adult?
12. Core Knowledge: Provider of Care	<u>Goals:</u> Recognize the benefits of interdisciplinary teams in care of older adults; evaluate the utility of complementary and integrative health practice on health promotion and symptom management <u>Example of a critical question to ask:</u> A. Are educational programs offered to health care staff about complementary and integrative health care for care of older adults?
13. Core Knowledge: Designer/Manager and Coordinator of Care	<u>Goals:</u> Facilitate older adults active participation in all aspects of their own health care; involve, educate and include significant others in implementing best practices for older adults; ensure quality of care commensurate with older adults vulnerability and frequency/intensity of care needs. <u>Examples of some critical questions to ask:</u> A. Does the team formerly assess or evaluate the older adults readiness to learn? or their ability to assimilate new information into their plan of care?
14. Core Knowledge: Member of a Profession	<u>Goals:</u> Promote quality preventive and end-of-life care for older adults as essential, desirable, and integral components of nursing practice. <u>Example of a critical question to ask:</u> A. Does the health care organization and team leaders educate its staff about illness prevention and/or how to provide quality end-of-life care?

References

Bloom, B. S. (Ed.). (1956). *Taxonomy of educational objectives: The classification of educational goals.* Chicago: Susan Fauer Company, Inc.

Delaware Valley Geriatric Education Center of the University of Pennsylvania. (2008). *TLC for LTC, teaching and learning for caregivers in long-term care.* Retrieved January 22, 2008, from http://www.nursing.upenn.edu/centers/hcgne/gero_tips/TLC/default.htm

Knowles, M. S. (1968). Androgogy, not pedagogy! *Adult Leadership, 16,* 350–352, 386.

Pennsylvania Intra-Governmental Council on Long Term Care. (2001). *In their own words: Pennsylvania's frontline workers in long-term care.* Author.

Leading Through Education in Long-Term Care Nursing

Post-test (circle one)

1. Name two characteristics of adult learners

   a. _____

   b. _____

Please circle the *best* answer among the items listed below.

Example:

This is a test.

   a. No, this is not a test.
   ⓑ Yes, this is a test.
   c. No, this is a joke.

The answer is ⓑ so it will be circled.

2. The education development process consists of:

   a. Needs assessment, objectives, design, and evaluation
   b. Needs assessment, teaching, reinforcement, and feedback
   c. Planning, delivery, and evaluation
   d. Planning, teaching objectives, delivery, and evaluation

3. Objectives are behavioral when they:

   a. Address behavior on the job
   b. Identify what the teacher will do
   c. Target what learners will be able to do
   d. Specify the domain of learning addressed

4. Needs assessment data appropriately include: (circle all that apply)

   a. Identified competencies/job description
   b. Focus groups
   c. Survey data
   d. Organization policies

189

e. Course outlines from professional meetings
f. Supervisor observations/reports
g. Quality Improvement data

5. Assumptions about adult learners include: (circle all that apply)

   a. Self-concept
   b. Experience
   c. Job level/position
   d. Readiness
   e. Motivation

6. The domains of learning include:

   a. Motivation, readiness, and self-concept
   b. Attitude, self-concept, and experience
   c. Skill, attitude, and readiness
   d. Knowledge, skill, and attitude

7. Teaching and learning experiences that might involve modifying a learner's attitudes include: (circle all that apply)

   a. Experiential or reflective
   b. Role play
   c. Crossword puzzles
   d. Perception exercise
   e. Exposing myths and stereotypes
   f. Demonstration

8. An example of an objective that involves learners mastering new information (knowledge) is:

   a. Manage personal feelings while caring for persons with dementia.
   b. Use a range of assessment strategies to identify the meaning of behavior.
   c. Individualize care to older adults with dementia to prevent and respond to behaviors.
   d. Discuss behavior as a form of communication.

9. Formative evaluation: (circle all that apply)

   a. Is when the cook tastes the soup.
   b. Sums up the program (person) with the aim of making decisions.

    c. Takes place while the program (person) is being formed with the aim of improvement.

    d. Is when the guests taste the soup.

10. The four levels of evaluation get progressively more challenging. Level 1: Reaction, measures the following:

    a. The impact of the educational program in relation to organizational needs and goals

    b. The ability of the learner to demonstrate acquisition of the knowledge, skills, or attitudinal objectives at the time of the program

    c. The ability of the learner to perform the cognitive, skill, and other objectives in the work

    d. How the learner felt about the program, how it met needs, and opinions about components of the program

Participant Evaluation Form

Leading Through Education in Long-Term Care Nursing

Today's Date ___/___/___   Facility: _____

Please circle the best response.

Example: Strongly Disagree   Disagree   Agree   Strongly Agree
                        1   2   3   4

At the end of the presentation I can:

1. Discuss the education development process: needs assessment, objectives, design and delivery, and evaluation.

Strongly Disagree   Disagree   Agree   Strongly Agree
          1   2   3   4

2. Discuss assumptions about adult learners in the long-term care workplace.

Strongly Disagree   Disagree   Agree   Strongly Agree
          1   2   3   4

3. Be more aware of how to conduct a needs assessment to gain a clear understanding of gaps in knowledge, desired skills, and shifts in attitudes.

Strongly Disagree   Disagree   Agree   Strongly Agree
          1   2   3   4

4. Discuss translation of needs into setting behavioral objectives.

Strongly Disagree   Disagree   Agree   Strongly Agree
          1   2   3   4

5. Discuss the domains of learning and different kinds of teaching and learning activities associated with each.

Strongly Disagree   Disagree   Agree   Strongly Agree
          1   2   3   4

6. Discuss the differences between formative evaluation and summative evaluation.

Strongly Disagree	Disagree	Agree	Strongly Agree
1	2	3	4

7. Identify strategies to apply the model, principles, and domains of learning into the long-term care setting.

Strongly Disagree	Disagree	Agree	Strongly Agree
1	2	3	4

8. This program will help me work better with clients/patients.

Strongly Disagree	Disagree	Agree	Strongly Agree
1	2	3	4

9. This program will help me work better with other staff.

Strongly Disagree	Disagree	Agree	Strongly Agree
1	2	3	4

Overall, I rate:

10. This program:

Poor	Fair	Good	Excellent
1	2	3	4

11. The interactive discussions:

Poor	Fair	Good	Excellent
1	2	3	4

12. Speaker _____ [insert name]

Poor	Fair	Good	Excellent
1	2	3	4

13. This program would be better if:

14. What other education-related topics would be helpful to you in the future?

Appendix

Pre- and Post-Test Answer Keys

Your ID _____   RN _____ Non RN _____
Today's Date ___/___/___   Facility: _____

Team Building
Pre/Post-Test Answer Key

Please circle the *best* answer among the items listed below.

Example:

This is a test.

  a. No, this is not a test.
  ⓑ Yes, this is a test.
  c. No, this is a joke.

The answer is ⓑ so it will be circled.

1. Senn, Childress, and Senn describe four styles of behavior in their self-scoring behavioral style/instrument. Which style is not described by this inventory?

  a. Controlling
  b. Promoting
  c. Judging*
  d. Analyzing

2. There are many characteristics of effective teamwork. What is the major requirement for effective teamwork?

  a. Respect
  b. Openness
  c. Empowerment
  d. Trust*

3. A team is

   a. An individual who is working on his/her own to accomplish a goal

   b. A group of people who are independent of each other but work to achieve a common group goal

   c. A group of people who are dependent on one another to achieve a common goal*

   d. None of the above

4. When working with someone with a controlling style, all of the following behaviors are effective EXCEPT:

   a. Spend time on the relationship before jumping to the task*

   b. Make your presentation stimulating and exciting

   c. Be decisive and self-confident

   d. Let them do most of the talking

5. Describe your behavioral style. (2 points)

6. Identify the strengths and weaknesses of your style. (4 points)

Your ID _____   RN _____ Non RN _____

Today's Date ___/___/___   Facility: _____

Directing and Delegation in Long-Term Care

Pre/Post-Test Answer Key

Please circle the *best* answer among the items listed below.

Example:

This is a test.

   a. No, this is not a test.

   (b.) Yes, this is a test.

   c. No, this is a joke.

The answer is (b) so it will be circled.

1. If you have delegated a task, you have momentarily transferred the responsibility of the task to _____?

   a. The delegatee*

   b. All the people on duty

   c. The charge nurse or nursing supervisor

   d. The delegator

2. If someone has delegated a task, _____ hold(s) the accountability of the task.

   a. The delegatee
   b. All the people on duty
   c. The charge nurse or nursing supervisor
   d. The delegator*

3. What must the delegator do for a new patient before assigning
   tasks to the delegatees?

   a. The delegator can assign any task to the delegatee if they
      are good friends and the delegator has been working with
      the delegatee for a long time.
   b. The delegator must assess the patient and make sure the
      task falls within the practice scope of the delegatee.*
   c. The delegator can assign any task to the direct care worker
      as long as the delegator trusts the direct care worker's
      judgment.
   d. When it is very busy, the RN delegator can ask the charge
      nurse (LPN) to carry out any nursing task, because the RN
      cannot be in two places at the same time.

4. Choose the letter that constitutes the five (5) rights of delegation from the information below:

   1. Right person
   2. Right thinking
   3. Right task
   4. Right circumstance
   5. Right shift
   6. Right supervision
   7. Right nursing home
   8. Right direction

   a. 1, 2, 4, 5, and 7
   b. 1, 3, 5, 7, and 8
   c. 1, 3, 4, 6, and 8*
   d. 1, 2, 5, 6, and 7

5. May the RN delegate the initial assessment of a patient with
   chest pain to an LPN?

   a. Yes, if the LPN has been working in the nursing home for
      10 years.
   b. Yes, if the LPN is attending classes to become a registered
      nurse.

    c.   No, because the patient is experiencing chest pain and initial assessment of chest pain must be done by an RN.*

    d.   Yes, if the LPN has been taking care of the patient longer than any other worker.

6.   The direct care worker is responsible for the initial assessment of the patient needs and must report findings to the RN as soon as possible.

    a.   Yes, the direct care worker knows the long term care resident the best.

    b.   No, the RN or LPN who is in charge has the responsibility of the initial assessment of the resident.*

    c.   No, because the patient may be having a chest pain, and initial assessment of chest pain must be done by an RN.

    d.   Yes, if the direct care worker is certified and attends a community college nursing program.

7.   The direct care worker is allowed to make nursing judgments if she has watched an LPN or RN care for another patient with similar experience in the past at the same facility.

    a.   Yes, because the direct care worker knows what is right for the residents.

    b.   No, because the RN or LPN are the only professionals who can make nursing judgments.*

    c.   No, because the residents may be having a chest pain, and initial assessment of chest pain must be done by an RN.

    d.   Yes, if the direct care worker is good and has been taking care of the resident for the longest amount of time.

8.   Does the RN need to supervise the direct care worker who has been working in the facility for a long time if the RN delegates a new task to that direct care worker?

    a.   No, because the direct care worker is usually certified.

    b.   No, because the RN or charge nurse is responsible for other services for the residents.

    c.   Yes, the direct care worker must be supervised for all tasks.

    d.   Yes, the RN or charge nurse must always supervise the direct care worker when delegating a new task that the direct care worker has not done before.*

9. In an urgent situation, in addition to assessing the patient, the RN/LPN is required to also assess the skill of the delegatee before delegation.

   a. Yes, because the direct care worker must be assessed to ensure competency.*
   b. No, if the RN heard that the direct care worker is an exceptional performer.
   c. No, because there is no time to do such assessment.
   d. No, if the direct care worker is certified.

10. As long as the task falls within the job description of the delegatee, the delegator is not accountable for the task.

    a. Yes, because the responsibility has been transferred.
    b. No, because the delegator will always be accountable even after delegating responsibility.*
    c. Yes, otherwise the purpose of delegation is defeated.
    d. Yes, especially if the delegatee is certified.

11. Conflict should always be avoided because it stops teamwork. (circle true or false)

    True   False*

12. Principal causes of conflict within organizations include which of the following:

    a. Misunderstandings, value and goal differences*
    b. Age differences
    c. Fluctuating leadership
    d. Level of education

13. Which of the following is not an appropriate conflict management mode (select one):

    a. Competing
    b. Collaborating
    c. Lying*
    d. Compromising
    e. Avoiding

14. When giving constructive feedback which of the following approaches is wrong (select one):

    a. Convey your positive intent.
    b. Make broad general statements rather than focus on specifics.*

    c.   State the impact of the behavior or action.

    d.   Ask the person to respond.

15. List two (2) action steps necessary to move from conflict to collaboration.

    a.   _____

    b.   _____

Mutual involvement; understand other person's point of view; keep conversation relevant; state the problem and its impact from your perspective; develop an appropriate plan of action; express appreciation of other person's point of view

_____

Your ID _____   RN _____ Non RN _____

Today's Date ___/___/___   Facility: _____

Power and Negotiation

Pre/Post–Test Answer Key

Please circle the *best* answer among the items listed below.

Example:

This is a test.

    a.   No, this is not a test.

    ⓑ   Yes, this is a test.

    c.   No, this is a joke.

The answer is ⓑ so it will be circled.

Power

1. Power is:

    a.   A characteristic that cannot be learned or acquired.

    b.   Viewed by many nurses to be immoral, corrupting, and contradictory to the caring nature of nursing.*

    c.   Strongest when it is given to an individual.

    d.   Not influenced by the situation.

2. Nurses may seek out another nurse who possesses expert knowledge about a clinical procedure. This is an example of what type of power?

    a. Legitimate power
    b. Referent power
    c. Reward power
    d. Expert power*

3. Middle power groups may do all of the following EXCEPT:

    a. Mediate between high and low groups
    b. Don't take risks in order to keep the favor of high power groups
    c. Withhold information and control communication*
    d. Get bought out by one or both groups

4. A strategy a nurse can use to develop a powerful image includes

    a. Use a phrase such as, "We have a problem."
    b. Take responsibility for communication.*
    c. Don't be flexible.
    d. Give little feedback to staff.

5. Describe how you plan to use power as an effective strategy in your workplace setting.

Negotiation

1. Negotiation is the art and science of:

    a. Creating agreements between two groups.*
    b. Establishing strategic alliances.
    c. Facilitating the participation of others in decisions.
    d. Pretending to be responsive to other's needs.

2. There are three approaches to negotiation, in the soft positional approach, the individual or group _____.

    a. Concede stubbornly
    b. Commit early; draft late
    c. Focus on interests, not positions
    d. Make threats

3. Positions and interests are important to identify in negotiations. The following are interests EXCEPT:

   a. Needs and concerns
   b. Terms and conditions*
   c. Fears and aspirations
   d. Underlying motivations

4. In negotiation, one needs to separate the process of *inventing* possible options for agreement from the process of *deciding among* those options. All of the following would be used as you try to *invent* possible options EXCEPT:

   a. Judging*
   b. Improving
   c. Generating
   d. Brainstorming

5. Give one example of effective use of negotiation strategies in your workplace setting.

   _____

Your ID _____   RN _____ Non RN _____
Today's Date ____/____/____   Facility: _____

Change Theory and Process

Pre/Post-Test Answer Key

Please circle T if the statement is True and F if the statement is False.

1. Everyone's initial response to change is anger.

   T   F*

2. Two requirements for effective individual change are willingness and anxiety related to potential job loss.

   T   F*

3. It is important for a leader to spend energy and time on all employees, especially those most resistant to change.

   T   F*

4. Individual responses to change can progress from denial to resistance to exploration and then commitment.

   T* F

5. When individuals are in a resistant mode it is important for the leader to continue to give them information and direction.

   T* F

6. During times of change, resilience is perceived as a negative attribute.

   T   F*

   Please circle the item that is not a characteristic.

7. To lead change a leader must be passionate, have a vision, and accept stumbles, falls, and move forward.

   T* F

8. Characteristics of change include all of the following EXCEPT:
   a. Evokes multiple responses
   b. It's inevitable and ever-present
   c. Slow paced and requires consensus*
   d. Can be disruptive, intrusive, and upsets status quo

   _____

Your ID _____   RN _____ Non RN _____
Today's Date ___/___/___   Facility: _____

Developing Cultural Competence in Long–Term Care Nursing
Pre/Post-Test Answer Key

Please circle the *best* answer among the items listed below.

1. Culturally competent care is best defined as:
   a. The use of one's personal experience to treat patients and staff.
   b. Using the institution's cultural staff to meet the needs of the patients and other staff.

    c. Understanding another culture that is different from one's own culture and using that knowledge to treat everyone else the same way.

    d. A set of skills, knowledge, and attitudes that respect the values of others when rendering care, even when it conflicts with one's own personal beliefs or values.*

2. Health care organizations need to provide culturally competent care because:

    a. It is documented in the Constitution of the United States.

    b. Many people cannot speak English or have limited proficiency in English.

    c. Of changing demographics, reports of health disparities, current legislative protocols, and evidence of positive patient outcomes.*

    d. Organizations will be able to receive more money from the government.

3. Cultural sensitivity is best described as:

    a. Being sensitive and respectful of the values and beliefs of others, which may or may not conflict with one's own values and beliefs.*

    b. Knowing that cultural differences and similarities exist within and between groups without assigning value to the differences.

    c. A process of changing one's personal values to those of others.

    d. Trying to learn another language so one can help the patients.

4. What is the first step to becoming a culturally competent health care provider?

    a. Talking with someone from another culture all the time.

    b. Self-appraisal of one's own cultural values and beliefs.*

    c. Listening and learning languages other than English.

    d. Taking classes to learn all the possible cultures in the world.

5. Choose the five strategies for bridging the cultural health gap, as outlined by Berlin and Fowkes.

    a. Assess, Explain, Evaluate, Implement, and Observe (AEEIO)

    b. Explain, Negotiate, Decide, Overcome, and Sign (ENDOS)

    c.   Listen, Explain, Acknowledge, Recommend, and Negotiate (LEARN)*

    d.   Assess, Decide, Implement, Evaluate, and Report (ADIER)

6. Which one of the following would not be an effective strategy for cross-cultural communication?

    a.   Having respect for the values of others

    b.   Seeing differences in others as primarily weaknesses*

    c.   Seeing differences as strengths rather than weaknesses

    d.   Recognizing unfamiliar situations as interesting instead of annoying

7. Communication about health beliefs and practices of residents/patients requires that culturally competent providers:

    a.   Discuss the meaning of health and illness, its etiology and cultural-specific concerns.

    b.   Provide opportunity for patients to describe their symptoms and approaches for coping with stressors.

    c.   Discuss the role of the family during sickness.

    d.   All of the above*

Match the following terms on the *left* to the correct definitions on the *right*.

Term		Definition
8. **Ethnicity**	_C_	A. Belief that race is the primary determinant of human traits and capabilities and the inherent superiority of a particular race.
9. **Stereotype**	_D_	B. Intentional or unintentional actions against a group or individuals based on gender, racial groups, ethnicity, sexual orientation, or education.
10. **Racism**	_A_	C. Self-defined affiliation with a specific group or subgroup that shares common cultural heritage due to history, customs, and language passed on from generation to generation.

11. **Discrimination** __B__   D. A fixed picture or set mental image that is used to represent all people from a group.

12. **Cultural**   __E__   E. Familiarization with cultural his-
    knowledge   tory, values, and belief systems of the members of another group.

Your ID _____   RN ____ Non RN ____
Today's Date ___/___/___   Facility: _____

Leading Through Education in Long-Term Care Nursing

Pre/Post-Test Answer Key

1. Name two characteristics of adult learners.

    a. self-concept, experience, readiness, problem-centered, motivation
    b. _____

Please circle the *best* answer among the items listed below.

Example:

This is a test.

    a. No, this is not a test.
    ⓑ Yes, this is a test.
    c. No, this is a joke.

The answer is ⓑ so it will be circled.

2. The education development process consists of:

    a. Needs assessment, objectives, design, and evaluation*
    b. Needs assessment, teaching, reinforcement, and feedback
    c. Planning, delivery, and evaluation
    d. Planning, teaching objectives, delivery, and evaluation

3. Objectives are behavioral when they:

    a. Address behavior on the job
    b. Identify what the teacher will do
    c. Target what learners will be able to do*
    d. Specify the domain of learning addressed

4. Needs assessment data appropriately include: (circle all that apply)

    a. Identified competencies/job description*
    b. Focus groups*
    c. Survey data*
    d. Organization policies*
    e. Course outlines from professional meetings
    f. Supervisor observations/reports*
    g. Quality Improvement data*

5. Assumptions about adult learners include: (circle all that apply)

    a. Self-concept*
    b. Experience*
    c. Job level/position
    d. Readiness*
    e. Motivation*

6. The domains of learning include:

    a. Motivation, readiness, and self-concept
    b. Attitude, self-concept, and experience
    c. Skill, attitude, and readiness
    d. Knowledge, skill, and attitude*

7. Teaching and learning experiences that might involve modifying a learner's attitudes include: (circle all that apply)

    a. Experiential or reflective*
    b. Role play*
    c. Crossword puzzles
    d. Perception exercise*
    e. Exposing myths and stereotypes*
    f. Demonstration

8. An example of an objective that involves learners mastering new information (knowledge) is:

    a. Manage personal feelings while caring for persons with dementia.
    b. Use a range of assessment strategies to identify the meaning of behavior.
    c. Individualize care to older adults with dementia to prevent and respond to behaviors.
    d. Discuss behavior as a form of communication.*

9. Formative evaluation: (circle all that apply)

    a.   Is when the cook tastes the soup.*

    b.   Sums up the program (person) with the aim of making decisions.

    c.   Takes place while the program (person) is being formed with the aim of improvement.*

    d.   Is when the guests taste the soup.

10. The four levels of evaluation get progressively more challenging. Level 1: Reaction, measures the following:

    a.   The impact of the educational program in relation to organizational needs and goals

    b.   The ability of the learner to demonstrate acquisition of the knowledge, skills, or attitudinal objectives at the time of the program

    c.   The ability of the learner to perform the cognitive, skill, and other objectives in the work

    d.   How the learner felt about the program, how it met needs, and opinions about components of the program*

Index

Made in the USA
Monee, IL
06 October 2020